FOREVER HOPE

First Edition, second printing.
First published in 2015
by Maida Vale Publishing
an imprint of Eyewear Publishing Ltd
Suite 38, 19-21 Crawford Street
London, WIH IPJ
United Kingdom

Graphic design by Edwin Smet
Author photograph by Christie Lacy Photography
Printed in England by TJ International Ltd, Padstow, Cornwall

Set in Auto 10,5 / 14,5 pt
ISBN 978-1-908998-47-7

FOREVER HOPE

Choosing Life Through Cancer and Recovery

By

LAURA SHOOK

OOO MAIDA VALE PUBLISHING

AN IMPRINT OF EYEWEAR PUBLISHING, LONDON, ENGLAND

2015

"Taste and see that the Lord is good.
Oh, the joys of those who take refuge
in Him!"
Psalm 34:8

PERMISSIONS

FOR MARK

"Across the years I will walk with you -
in deep green forests; on shores of sand:
and when our time on earth is through,
in heaven, too, you will have my hand"

Robert Sexton

PREFACE

I started writing about my cancer journey in a private journal. I quickly realized that my kids would need regular updates since they all lived away from home, so I turned my journal into an online blog. Finally, overwhelmed with the number of people in our circle of family and friends who wanted to know how to pray for us, I made that blog public. It became a daily comfort for me to sit quietly with God and document all that he was teaching me. For several years I have been encouraged to share my story with a wider audience. I never intended to write a book. Being an author was never something I have aspired to. But, after so many fellow cancer strugglers and their families shared with me the courage and strength they received from the story of my cancer journey, I told the Lord I was open and available to do whatever He wanted me to do in this regard.

In April, 2013, I was eating breakfast in a small cafe in Paris, France with my husband Mark, our son David and his wife Syd, and David's publisher Dr. Todd Swift, the owner of Eyewear Publishing. We were celebrating the debut of David's first book of poetry (*Our Obsidian Tongues*). In the course of that conversation, Dr. Swift began to talk about publishing books from a Christian perspective and David said, right out loud, "My mom has a book." I was surprised by his statement. I smiled, graciously acknowledged David's kind words, and waited to move on to other subjects. But the publisher was intrigued. "Have you really written a book?" he asked. "I am very interested in publishing books related to spirituality, and I would very much like to see what you've written." I told him I was a cancer survivor. Within the next five minutes of conversation, he was ready to commit to publish my story. I encouraged him to read it first, and then we could talk. By the time we arrived home, I had an email from the publisher waiting for me. He was serious. I was still unsure about the prospect. Then one day, as I prayed, God reminded me of our earlier conversation. So this book is His doing.

INTRODUCTION

One of my editors asked me to write a little of the back-story as an introduction to this book. But here's the thing – cancer has no back-story. It strikes suddenly, out of nowhere, with no consideration of persons. Everyone I know tried to figure out why I had cancer. Surely I must have had certain risk factors, or some sort of family history of the disease. None of those things were true of me. According to the American Cancer Society's website nearly 1.6 million people in the U.S. alone will be diagnosed with cancer this year. Cancer is an invader. And it's relentless. That's the only back-story.

But into that grim picture, steps hope. Through the mercy and grace of a loving God, I found the cancer journey to not only be survivable, but to be a source of incredible growth, unimaginable joy, and an experience I will forever be grateful to have lived to tell.

My story began in 2009 when my doctor spoke the word "cancer" to me for the first time. Unfortunately, he spoke "cancer" and *my* name in the same sentence, setting me on a path I never could have imagined. Writing has always been my way of processing emotions, whether love, fear, angst, joy, or heartache, so it was natural to write about my experience. What follows is the play-by-play of cancer. It's my daily journal - honest, heartfelt, and intense. I hope through the telling of my very personal, detailed journey, you will see the goodness of God. And to the cancer warriors who find their way to these pages, I want you to know that you are not alone. I pray my story will encourage you along the way and bring you hope in the chaos.

You can get through this too!

I firmly believe that God has been orchestrating my life from before the time that I was born. Not because I am special in any way, but solely because that's who He is – a compassionate Father. I grew up in a loving home with my parents and two brothers, Steve and Cary. God blessed me with the husband of my dreams, Mark, and filled my life with overflowing love when he gave me three children, David, Sarah, and Ashley, and their spouses. He has allowed us to live a crazy, adventure-filled life, leaving our footprints all across the globe. We have served together on several church staffs, and served as missionaries in Costa Rica and Mexico. In 2003 we founded Community of Faith in Houston, Texas. It has grown to be one of the largest churches in the nation, but at the same time it is a place that is full of a spirit of love and acceptance that is transformational. I am so thankful that God knew I would need to be in this place on that day in May when my life turned upside down.

*

"Laura has faced the giant. I am reminded of the words David spoke as he faced Goliath, '*The Lord does not deliver by sword or by spear; for the battle is the Lord's and He will give you into our hands.*'(1 Sam. 17:47)

This book chronicles her battle with the same faith in our powerful God. Laura peels back the curtain and lets her reader observe the details of her fight. All said, this is an intimate story of faith that ends with victory!"
– *Dr. Ed Young, Senior Pastor,*
Second Baptist Church, Houston, Texas

*

"Laura Shook's book is a moving testimony of hope and trust in the God of all hope. It is written with grace, humor, honesty, and the kind of faith that endures in the midst of doubt and fear.

The entire time I was reading I noticed several things: One, that it was beautifully written. Two, that in some ways I felt the main character was God, not even Laura, whose utter honesty about the emotions she felt in dealing with her cancer challenged and stirred my own trust and faith. Third, I could feel Laura's internal and deeply personal struggles, and while God was the subject, the cast of characters included more than just Laura – it included her family, her church, and people all over the world.

You normally don't think of words like 'submission' and 'choosing to fight' in the same context; but, I felt all of those things in reading Laura's faithful, submissive, and honest testimony to the power of God in the midst of a personal, health catastrophe.

This is a powerful testimony of faith, and I highly recommend it for anyone who has just received a diagnosis of cancer."
– *Dr. Robert Sloan, President,*
Houston Baptist University

*

"Laura Shook has written a book that is unsparingly honest, deeply personal, and extraordinarily courageous. As a self-confessed 'introvert,' she could have decided to turn inward upon learning that she had cancer, falling back into anger, pessimism, and self-pity. Instead she chose to share her experiences with other sufferers and their families – bringing faith, strength, love, perseverance, and even humor to her ordeal and to the many lives she has touched and will touch with this book. Regardless of your own personal circumstance, *Forever Hope* will inspire you to live every day to the fullest, to take nothing for granted, and to always appreciate those you love and who love you."

–Thomas J. Donohue, President & CEO,
U.S. Chamber of Commerce

*

"Having led Marines into the 'Valley of the Shadow of Death,' I thought I knew a little about courage, faith, and strength of character. I then read Laura Shook's remarkable book, *Forever Hope*, and realized that Marines have no "lock" on those traits. Laura expertly brings the reader into her world of fear and faith, of battling and believing, and finally into understanding the power of prayer and the healing hand of God. I could not put the book down!"

- Charles C. Krulak, General, USMC (Ret.)
31st Commandant of the Marine Corps

*

"In *Forever Hope*, Laura Shook opens her life and heart as she shares about her battle with cancer. She is a transparent storyteller who takes us on her journey with humor, honesty, and hope. Through it all, she never loses sight of God's plan for her life. Readers dealing with serious illnesses will be touched by Laura's inspiring courage."

– Mac McQuiston, President and CEO, CEO Forum

*

"The book, *Forever Hope*, written by Laura Shook, really hits home with anyone who has been diagnosed with cancer or has a family member dealing with that very frightening illness. It's a word no one wants to hear, but her story really shows that you can attain great strength and courage from our Lord, and that He will help you through it."

– Drayton McClane Chairman and CEO, McLane Group
and Former Owner of the Houston Astros

DIAGNOSIS

"Faith is finally this:
resting so utterly in the character of God
– in the ultimate goodness of God –
that you trust him even when he
seems untrustworthy."

Mark Buchanan

Wednesday May 27, 2009
Life Interrupted

This is the day I learn I have cancer. Weird. I never thought I'd hear those words, especially not today. I am still drowsy from anesthesia. The doctor just comes in, and she says, "Well, we thought it was hemorrhoids, but it's not. It's a tumor. It's cancer." Just like that. Now I am a person with cancer.

March 2009, I start bleeding. It's never happened before in my life. I assume it's hemorrhoids and wait for it to go away. But something just doesn't feel right. And it doesn't go away. I had a breast biopsy in April and that freaked me out. It made me start to pay attention to my body. I happened to see Dr. Oz on Oprah one day. It was his last time to be on her show, and they brought on several people to thank Dr. Oz and explain to him how he saved their life. One lady said she went to get a colonoscopy because Dr. Oz once mentioned on the show that everyone over the age of fifty should get a colonoscopy. She had cancer. No symptoms. Dr. Oz saved her life.

I see repeated advertisements on TV for Farrah Fawcett's documentary about her cancer journey. A member of our church is suddenly diagnosed with colon cancer and it has already spread to his lymph nodes, just like that, suddenly.

During this time, I start waking up in the nights with praise music playing in my head, lyrics about God being in control, about His answering when I call out in the night, over and over again. I begin to wonder what God is telling me, feeling like He is preparing me for something to come.

So, I decide to see a doctor. It's probably hemorrhoids, but better to die of embarrassment than to die of cancer. Problem is I don't have a personal physician. I haven't needed one; I'm never sick. The first doctor I call can't see me until July, and I discover it's hard to find a doctor with available appointments. The bleeding motivates me to find someone who can see me sooner rather than later. I spend all afternoon stressed over choosing a doctor. I finally call one I found on the Internet because I like how their webpage looks. Admittedly not the best way to choose a doctor, but that's the world we live in, right? I whisper a prayer, "God, if you want me to see this doctor, please show me," and I dial the number. I easily get an appointment to see the doctor the following week, on my daughter Sarah's 21st birthday. God heard my prayer.

In spite of my misgivings, the first appointment was easy. Much to my relief, no internal physical exam is required. The doctor tells me that at my age, ninety-nine percent of the time it is internal hemorrhoids or polyps. They schedule a colonoscopy for the following week.

I debate having this procedure all week. So much else is going on. Our daughter Ashley is getting ready to graduate from high school. We are getting ready to take a group from our church to Africa. I don't really have time to have cancer; maybe I should put it off. Then I start doing the colon prep for the colonoscopy. God help me! I can't drink this stuff without gagging. Finally I get it done, there is nothing left in my system. On the morning of the colonoscopy, we find a seat in the waiting room. It's a busy place and the wait is long.

I am sitting in a room full of elderly people, wondering what I'm doing here. How can this be my life? I am never sick. Then they roll me into the room for the procedure. The nurse turns on soft music, and I recognize the song. "Our God Reigns" is playing. This is how I fall asleep. My God reigns.

I wake up a cancer patient. My husband, Mark, asks the doctor to repeat the news four times. *Are you sure?* Somehow hoping that she will change her mind if he just asks once more.

The nurse brings me two bottles of banana flavored liquid barium to drink. It is just like liquid chalk. Honestly, after forty-eight hours of a clear liquid diet, it tastes pretty good! I am wheeled into another room to have a CT scan. *They are checking the rest of my body for cancer. Can this really be happening? I feel like I have entered some sort of time warp and been transported to the Twilight Zone.* They make plans for me to come back the next day for another colonoscopy and an ultrasound. I am sent home with instructions not to eat – clear liquids only. I am already sick of Jell-O and this is only the beginning.

Later, at home, I am getting ready to go see one of my favorite musicals, *Fiddler on the Roof.* The tickets were my Christmas present to my parents. Everyone wonders why we're still going, but it's better than sitting at home feeling hungry, right? And besides, are we going to let "cancer" run our life?

The phone rings – the CT scan is clean, no spread of the tumor. I am on the floor of the shower, facedown, crying in praise to my God who is merciful – Grateful that you hear and understand the groaning of my spirit when words won't come. Thank you.

Thursday May 28, 2009

Day two of cancer. It is Ashley's last day of high school. The last time I'll wake her up singing, "School days, school days, happy golden rule days!" The last time I'll spend the quiet morning with her, making her breakfast and making sure she has what she needs for school. Life is strange. I guess God gave me something else to think about instead of dwelling on the fact that Ashley will be leaving for college soon and my whole life is changing - daily motherhood is over.

It's a beautiful day outside. God sent a cool morning with a pretty sunrise. I whisper a prayer. Thank you that you are here.

Thank you for waking me up with music in my head. Thank you that you are the God of the universe and you are ruling on your eternal throne. Thank you that you are *Jehovah Rapha*, the God who heals.

Today will be another fun day of colonoscopy with ultrasound. Lord, please be peace and strength for my husband, my children, and my parents. Please don't let my parents suffer the grief of losing a child.

I sit down to read my Bible before we head to the doctor's office today and this is what I read:

"The Lord will fight for you; you need only to be still." Exodus 14:14 (NIV)

I immediately know it is God speaking. I am flooded with a supernatural peace. He will be with me as I lie on the stretcher today and suffer the humiliation of a second colonoscopy and an internal ultrasound. He will strengthen me today.

An email from a friend says, "God has trusted your family with this crisis," and I am encouraged by that perspective.

I know we have to let our church staff and our closest friends know what's going on. Without their prayer support we'll never make it through this chaos. Email seems to be the quickest way to get the news out.

My dear sweet friends,

My guess is you have probably already heard this news, but just in case, I am sending you this email. I'm sorry to send this news to you in an email, but it is the fastest way to let you all know.

I had a colonoscopy yesterday for what I thought was probably just internal hemorrhoids... but the news was not that good. I have a rectal tumor that the doctor says is most likely cancer. The biopsy won't be back until Friday, but she was pretty certain that it is cancer. The good news is that after they found the tumor they did a CT scan to see if it had already spread to any other organs or the lymph nodes and they didn't find any evidence of the cancer anywhere else. I didn't know I could feel so happy about anything on the day I was told I had cancer, but that was pretty happy news!

This morning they are going to do another type of colonoscopy with ultrasound to determine how deep into the wall of the colon the tumor is. This will help determine the severity of the disease. From there, I guess we'll be going to visit a surgeon and oncologist next week.

Most of you are probably reading this in the morning, and I'm sorry to start your day off with this news. But I really need you to pray for me. Please pray for healing, and for wisdom as we walk this road. And please pray especially for Mark, our kids, David, Sydneyann, Sarah, and Ashley, and my parents. I think this has been more shocking for them than it has been for me.
I love you guys! God is still on His throne!

Laura

Friday May 29, 2009

It's so weird how time keeps going. I've always seen that to be true in times of crisis or disaster, but it's interesting to experience it firsthand. I HAVE CANCER! ...And life goes on.

Many tears today – for Mark, for my kids, for my parents, for my friends, for plans that must change, for sweet, sweet emails from my friends. I love you all!

What do I say now, when someone casually asks, "Hey, how are you?" "I'm good!" or "Fine." don't seem like appropriate responses, but neither does, "I have cancer." As I contemplate what my response should be, I am struck with this truth. I really am fine. Really, nothing has changed from two days ago – God is still on His throne. He is still good. He is still in control. He is still working out His good plans just like He was two days ago. I'm good. Really.

I have an appointment to get my hair done today and I wonder, will I have hair when it's time to go back to see my hairdresser, Patricia, in a couple of months? And how do I tell her? *How do I tell anyone?*

The tears come again... Oh God, please help me to trust you. I can see I need to invest in waterproof mascara!

Saturday May 30, 2009

Mark did a great job tonight sharing with Community of Faith all that is going on. I didn't even really cry, just sat on the front row and shook the whole time. Our worship leader and good friend Donald picked some of my favorite praise songs to sing. Mom, Dad, and my brother Cary were there. They told me that when Mark started reading my journal Daddy laid his head on Mom's shoulder weeping. I'm glad I didn't see that, it would have been the end for me.

I dropped a bowl with cat food in it tonight and I lost it – I'm mad at the pets, as if they've done something wrong. I don't want to be this person! I don't want to be the person with cancer. I don't want my plans to be messed up. Everything was going so well. Mark and I just spent the last week talking about our life and how everything was getting ready to change. We will have an empty nest. We were making plans for next steps at the church and our work around the world. Everything is on hold now and I'm angry at the cat.

My prayer for my life, my family's life, and for Community of Faith at the beginning of the year was that we would all say, I am yours, body and soul. Like Mary, Jesus' mother, said in response to God's call on her life. I've been praying that for months. Little did I know it would be my own life where I would see my faith challenged and stretched. You must have been smiling as I prayed, God, you knew.

Sunday May 31, 2009

I wake up with music in my head again today, Chris Tomlin singing *Worthy is the Lamb*.

"And I hear the voice of many angels sing, 'Worthy is the Lamb', I hear the cry of every longing heart, 'Worthy is the Lamb' ("I Will Rise," by Chris Tomlin, et.al.).

I join them in singing!

I've met a lot of cancer survivors over the past two days – I am counting myself among them! It has been sweet to experience the Body of Christ in action, living as God intended, loving as God commanded. It's crazy to see God orchestrating my life!

Last Thursday a very dear friend called out of the blue. She had no idea that I had been diagnosed with cancer. She was calling to tell me that her breast cancer was back...we talked, cried, and laughed together. She has been down this road before. It was so good to hear from someone who understands what I am feeling and experiencing.

Our good friend Derek came to the house and hung out for a while – Derek is the kind of guy you can make cancer jokes with and he doesn't freak out. It felt so good to laugh!

Later Donald came by the house to finalize plans for the weekend worship services. Donald's mother fought a 16-year battle with breast cancer when he was in high school and college. What an incredible gift to have someone on our side who has walked this path before, who understands how Mark is feeling, and who is fiercely protective of us.

My nieces and nephew, Sydney, Chandler and Bryce stood by

my side this weekend as we shared our news with the church. Their presence gave me strength, and it also deepened my motivation to fight this thing.

I feel like I am in a safe place. I know God has put these people around us to strengthen us. I know they have our backs and I am so grateful.

"He comes alongside us when we go through hard times, and before you know it, he brings us alongside someone else who is going through hard times so that we can be there for that person just as God was there for us." 2 Corinthians 1:4 (The Message)

Monday June 1, 2009

It feels like there are two of me, the "Normal Laura" that performs the everyday tasks of life, and the "Cancer Patient Laura" who is consumed by doctor appointments, medical procedures, phone calls, waiting, and fear.

Each Monday morning I go into "Cancer Patient Laura" mode. Fear is a constant companion. It permeates everything, just under the surface. Fear of the unknown. Fear for my children. Fear of the future. Fear that I won't be able to handle what comes my way. But then I remember that faith is not the absence of fear, faith is choosing to trust God in spite of the fear I feel. That's it – faith is a choice.

How many times have I taught that lesson? Faith is a choice. Choose faith today, Laura. I look back at all the Ladies Bible Studies I've taught just this year. Every one was centered on the fact that we have to choose. God gave those lessons for ME!

Just last month I shared these Scripture verses while teaching the Ladies Bible Study at the church:

"Pour out your heart to God, for He is our refuge." Psalm 62:8 (NLT)

"'In my distress, I said, God cannot see me!' But you heard my

prayer when I cried out to you for help." Psalm 31:22 (NCV)

"…We saw how powerless we were to help ourselves; but that was good for then we put everything into the hands of God, who alone could save us, for He can even raise the dead." 2 Corinthians 1:9 (TLB)

"So we're not giving up. How could we! Even though on the outside it often looks like things are falling apart on us, on the inside, where God is making new life, not a day goes by without his unfolding grace." 2 Corinthians 4:16 (The Message)

Every verse intended for me! Thank you, God for your words!

Today we visited the colorectal surgeon, an experience I hope to never repeat! The surgeon and his staff were all extremely kind. He spent over an hour with us answering all of our questions. Then he asked, "Would you like me to examine you?" I had no idea what I was getting into. I was taken to an exam room with a strange looking table in the middle of the room. It is L-shaped with a short, flat padded surface and another padded surface going down the side that ends in a kneeler. The nurse gently asked me to drop my pants and kneel, leaning over the table. I am mortified. Every other exam I have endured to this point has thankfully been performed under the mind numbing power of anesthesia. This is different. She covers my back side with a paper drape and in that position I wait for the surgeon to enter the room.

The surgeon arrives and snaps on his latex gloves. With his headlamp in place, he grabs a rubber tube for the purpose of pumping air into my rectum. He activates the foot pedal and suddenly the table is moving. My head drops toward the floor, my bottom rises in the air. I hold onto the table for life, squeeze my eyes shut as tightly as I can to prevent the tears from falling to the floor; and I desperately pray. Again I wonder how this could be my life, how I ended up on a motorized table with my pants at my ankles while someone looks into my bowels. Is this real life? "Jesus, Jesus, Jesus," I plead silently in my head. "I can't do this. I need you," I pray, as the surgeon takes a punch biopsy of the tumor. I wonder if this irritation of the invader will release cancer cells into the rest of my body. I have no idea if that's how cancer operates, but I wonder if my fate is sealed in this moment.

Note to self: Always bring an extra pair of pants when you are going to visit the colorectal surgeon. You never know when you might need them!

The surgeon sends me to the medical center in downtown Houston. There, the plan is to perform another internal ultrasound of the tumor to get a better picture of what's going on. I silently follow instructions. I completely shut down my brain and emotions as I climb onto another exam table and allow three new doctors to do their thing. By this point, nothing can embarrass me anymore.

While I am waiting to pay my bill, I overhear the doctor who performed the ultrasound give his report to my surgeon over the phone. I'm sure I am not supposed to hear that conversation, but I stay in position, eavesdropping until the doctor hangs up. I hear him say "three lymph nodes." My heart sinks; my legs feel weak. I hope I will be able to walk out to the car. Mark drives me home and I don't have the heart to tell him what I heard.

Later that afternoon, the surgeon calls and tells us what I already overheard. The second ultrasound does show that three lymph nodes are involved and the tumor has already broken through the wall of the rectum and grown into the surrounding fat tissue. If the biopsy shows cancer cells, then we are looking at chemotherapy and radiation in the near future, and surgery within the next three months. If they don't find any cancer cells then it will be a very unusual tumor and they will take out larger sections of the tumor to be able to study it more. I have a PET scan scheduled for Wednesday to check the whole body for cancer cells.

I sink into the couch, exhausted, defeated, numb. God where are you? Then the words of author Mark Buchanan enter my mind:

> "Faith is finally this: resting so utterly in the character of God - in the ultimate goodness of God - that you trust him even when he seems untrustworthy."

God, please help me to remember who you are.

Night Watch

4:30 a.m. Music in my head: "Yesterday, today, and forever, you are the same, you never change. Yesterday, today, and forever, you are faithful and I will trust in you!" ("Yesterday, Today, and Forever," by Vickie Beeching)

I keep waking up early in the morning. I decide to use this time to pray for my cancer partners, those friends I personally know who are also fighting cancer – Mary, Bruce, John, Kevin, and Roosevelt. God please bring miraculous healing to their bodies. Please meet their physical needs today as they endure medical tests and procedures, receive radiation, chemotherapy, and recover from surgery. Please strengthen their immune systems; please give them your wisdom as they make decisions about their doctors and treatment. Please help them choose to trust you today. Please meet the needs of their family members and those who love them. Please give them your supernatural peace and strength and courage for whatever the day holds. Help them to recognize your presence today, and to hear your voice. Wrap them up in your arms. Teach them, grow them, make them, stretch them, use them. Glorify yourself in each of these sweet friends, so that they, in turn, may glorify you. God heal them.

Tuesday June 2, 2009

I am one of those people who like to have a schedule, like to keep a calendar, like to make lists and check things off. Obviously the past week has really blown my schedule to pieces!

The first thing I thought when I was told of the tumor was, "But I'm going to Africa!"

My first all-important question for the surgeon was not a medical question. I asked him, "I am supposed to leave for Africa next week and be gone for a month. What do you think about that?"

Of course he smiled and said, "You need to just go ahead and cancel those plans. Let's get you well first."

I don't take kindly to having my plans messed up! In fact it made me a little angry! I was having a conversation with God about this situation the other day and it went something like this:

"I am supposed to go to Africa in June! And I'm going with the church group to Costa Rica in July! And I'm going to my nephew's wedding in August! And we're moving Ashley to college soon. You can't just come in here and mess up all my plans! I mean, who do you think you are anyway? God??"

– Silent pause –

"Oh, yeah, you ARE God. I guess maybe your plans are better than my plans."

This revelation led to the exchange of my calendar and my plans for God's. I know His plans for me are perfect.

A sweet friend wrote this recently and it stuck with me: "So many times God has denied me the desires of my heart only to provide me with the needs of my soul." And I think that's what He's doing now in my life.

We received the report of the second biopsy today. They found cancer cells. I will have the PET scan tomorrow to check the rest of the body for cancer cells. I will go see a radiologist and oncologist at the end of the week.

"'For I know the plans I have for you,' says the Lord. 'They are plans for good and not for disaster, to give you a future and a hope.'" Jeremiah 29:11 (NLT)

Wednesday June 3, 2009

Waiting seems to be the operative word when it comes to cancer diagnosis and treatment. This is something I will have to learn to do.

No news today. I had the PET scan done and we are waiting for the report. It is interesting to enter a small room with a huge radiation warning sign on the door! The technician mixes the glucose injection in a huge lead box. He comes to me with a syringe surrounded by an inch thick lead casing and proceeds to inject this substance into my body. Makes you wonder, if I didn't have cancer before, will I have it now?

One of the most amazing things has been to watch the Body of Christ in action! So many people are praying for me around the globe that God is probably tired of hearing about me! Thousands of people have heard my name or read my story in the past week. New friends, old friends, and people I've never met are praying for me. Adults are praying for me, students are praying for me, children are praying for me. How amazing is that? Literally, tens of thousands of people are praying for me. Wow! Thank you, God, for the way you designed your body, the church, to work! What a beautiful symphony this must be in your ears!

So far, I know that I am being prayed for in Australia, Korea, England, Afghanistan, Burundi, Venezuela, Costa Rica, Dominican Republic, Haiti, Mexico, Canada, and the United States. A constant intercession on my behalf! I know God is going to do incredible things in answer to these prayers! I am humbled by this kindness and grateful for the faithfulness of so many.

My brother Cary has started a 24/7 prayer chain for me called "Laura's Symphony of Prayer." He is hoping to fill up ten-minute time slots around the clock of people around the world praying for me. I have the two best brothers in the world!

I read this verse today: *"I have cared for you since before you were born. I will be your God throughout your lifetime - until your hair is white with age. I made you, and I will care for your. I will carry you along and save you." Isaiah 46:3b-4 (NLT)*

Thank you, God, that you are carrying me along on the prayers of so many.

Thursday June 4, 2009
Good News!

After several days of progressive bad news, we finally received good news today! The PET scan did not show any spread of the cancer! The cancer was seen in the one tumor and in only one lymph node beside it! This is amazingly good news! It is still considered a stage three cancer and will be treated with the three-prong protocol of radiation, chemotherapy, and surgery. We met with the radiation oncologist today who explained all about radiation therapy to us. I'm not sure how much of what he explained I actually absorbed, but here is what I know so far. He plans to do 28 days of radiation combined with oral chemotherapy. Monday through Friday, five days a week, for

28 days. There are some common side effects of this treatment including fatigue, nausea, cramping, and diarrhea. He told me to invest in Gatorade. This all sounds eerily similar to my experience with the colon-cleansing project. I'm looking forward to some interesting days ahead.

We will meet with the medical oncologist tomorrow afternoon to learn all the fun facts about chemotherapy (*said with a small dose of sarcasm*).

Following the weeks of radiation and chemotherapy I will get a 4-6 week break to heal and then have surgery to remove the tumor. Everything we are doing now is to decrease the probability of a recurrence of cancer in the future or the "seeding" of cancer cells in the surgical site. The idea is to kill the cancer cells before the surgery.

The good news is I am now the proud owner of a "Radiation Therapy Parking Permit" and my very own Radiation Therapy bar code check-in card! Not everyone can say they have those. The bad news is I will not be able to swim or sit in the Jacuzzi during the weeks of radiation treatment. How will I survive a Houston summer without the pool?

Song in my head today: "All my delight is in you Lord. All of my hope, and all of my strength." ("None But Jesus," by Brooke Gabrielle Fraser)

"But you, O Lord, are a shield around me; my glory, and the one who holds my head high. I cried out to the Lord, and he answered me from his holy mountain. I lay down and slept, yet I woke up in safety, for the Lord was watching over me... Victory comes from you O Lord. May you bless your people." Psalm 3:3-5 & 8 (NLT)

Friday June 5, 2009
Stop the World I Want to Get Off

Nine days ago I discovered I have cancer. So much has happened in such a short time. My emotions are pretty volatile. Most of the time I am calm and have such a sense of God's peace and His protection about me. Then suddenly I am angry, or extremely irritable, or grieving and crying. The littlest things can set me off on one of these emotional breaks. I am not sure how to manage my normal life when something so all consuming has taken over.

I am an introvert. I need time alone to process, to recuperate, to restore my soul. The past nine days I have been overwhelmed with people – doctors, nurses, technicians, accounts payable, pharmacists, lab techs, friends, family members, and phone calls. I try to remember that cancer is a "family" illness, but sometimes I want to scream, "I am the one who is sick here! Can you all just get away from me and leave me alone?" I have been poked and prodded, and probed way too many times in unimaginable ways. People casually discuss my private body functions. I know they do this every day, but I don't.

Truthfully, I am grateful for their knowledge, skill, and expertise. I am grateful for their compassion toward me, and their desire to see me well. But I am very tired of people. Right now I just want to crawl in my bed and hide from the world.

In my short experience with cancer I have found that cancer doctors, cancer nurses, and cancer patients are the kindest people I have ever met, seriously. I hope people will be able to say this of me too.

Today I went back to the radiation oncologist to have my simulation done. This is the process where they measure my body and mark my skin to show where the radiation beams will be directed. They also made a custom immobilization device for me that will be used to hold me in the exact position each time I receive radiation.

During the simulation, I was lying on the radiation table and was overcome with emotion. Reality seems to break through in tiny spurts; I guess because God knows that's all I can handle at once. What am I doing here? How can this be my life? This is all so surreal. I start to cry. The nurse brings me a tissue and reassures me. They begin to move the table into the radiation machine and tell me to remain still. How can I be still when I'm about to start sobbing? Focus, Laura, breathe deep, God is here. So I begin to sing "Jesus Loves Me" to myself. Not out loud or they will hear me on the intercom. I am mouthing the words over and over. I sing all the songs I used to sing to my children when they were babies. Keeping my focus on Jesus. He is here. I can do this.

"Let us fix our eyes on Jesus, the author and perfecter of our faith, who for the joy set before him endured the cross, scorning its shame, and sat down at the right hand of the throne of God." Hebrews 12:2 (NIV)

"…whenever trouble comes your way, let it be an opportunity for joy. For when your faith is tested, your endurance has a chance to grow. So let it grow, for when your endurance is fully developed, you will be strong in character and ready for anything." James 1:2 (NLT)

Saturday June 6, 2009
His Mercies Are New Every Morning

The song in my head and heart today:
"All that is within me cries for you alone.
Be glorified.
Emmanuel, God with us.
My heart sings a brand new song.
The debt is paid, these chains are gone.
Emmanuel, God with us."
("God With Us," by Barry Graul, et.al.)

Thank You, Lord, for a good night's sleep and a brand new day. Thank You that our daughter Sarah is home. Her presence brings me strength.

Yesterday we met with the medical oncologist. I liked him. He was very positive and encouraging. His whole staff was very supportive. His plan is to start me on oral chemotherapy beginning Monday to go along with the radiation. The two enhance each other in my case when used simultaneously. It will be a moderate dose of chemotherapy and the doctor expects minimal side effects. That's good news! No hair loss, only mild nausea and fatigue. The biggest problem I can expect is diarrhea as a result of the radiation. I have been told that within a couple of weeks I will want to stay close to a bathroom at all times! This will last up to six weeks. He also said that with this dose of chemotherapy my immune system will not be compromised like it is with higher doses – more good news! I can still see and hug everyone at Community of Faith!

Radiation and chemotherapy will be Monday through Friday. I will get good use of my parking pass as I make daily trips to the radiation center!

"Because of the Lord's great love we are not consumed, for his compassions never fail. They are new every morning; great is your faithfulness." Lamentations 3:22-23 (NIV)

Sunday June 7, 2009
Glory, Honor, and Power Belong to You!

I spent Saturday afternoon reading. We have received so much material from doctors, pharmacists, treatment centers and other places I felt like I needed to read everything before we actually get started on treatment. Now I feel confident that we have made the right decisions about doctors, hospitals, and treatment.

I believe that we are in good hands.

A lot of this material includes numbers: five-year survival rates, prognosis numbers, chance of recurrence, and many others. The numbers can be scary when you read about rectal cancer. They don't look particularly good.

And then God reminded me...

"You saw me before I was born. Every day of my life was recorded in your book. Every moment was laid out before a single day had passed. " Psalm 139:16 (NLT)

God decided how many days I would live before I was ever born. This cancer has absolutely no impact on how long I will live. It can't shorten my life. God has already numbered my days. This is a very comforting thought for me. My life has always been in God's hands. Cancer is not in control, God is. Glory, honor, and power belong to Him! Thank You, Lord, that You are my God.

TREATMENT

"You gain strength, courage, and confidence
by every experience in which you really stop to look fear in the
face. You are able to say to yourself, 'I have lived through this
horror. I can take the next thing that comes along'...
You must do the thing you cannot do."

Eleanor Roosevelt

Monday June 8, 2009
1 Down, 27 To Go

Day One of Treatment. I woke up nervous, still coming to grips with the reality of what is going on in my life. But as soon as we started treatment it felt really good to actually be doing something about "Bob" the tumor. Yes, he has a name. We considered other names, some of them not so pretty, but in the end just decided to go with something simple. To all you Bobs out there, sorry, this is no reflection on you.

I took three pills this morning after breakfast, had a radiation treatment at 2:00 and took three more pills after dinner. This will be the plan for the next six weeks. I did wear my "chemo sweatband" as well as my "I am going to beat cancer" socks to radiation. The sweatband was a gift from Ashley, and the socks were a gift from a friend. Somehow it gives me courage to have them with me for my treatments, reminding me that many are praying for my healing.

We are all praying specifically that the medication and radiation will do exactly what they are supposed to do; praying for protection of normal healthy cells and destruction of cancer cells; and praying for minimal side effects - you know what I'm talking about!

Monday June 9, 2009
The Power of Human Touch

I am a registered nurse. When I was in nursing school I remember studying the healing power of touch. I never fully understood it until now.

I was on the exam table in the office of the colorectal surgeon, in a very uncomfortable position, enduring a very uncomfortable exam. The nurse reached out and touched my arm. It was a very small gesture, but it spoke volumes to me. That touch instantly transmitted peace to me. It told me that they recognized I was still a person and not just a cancer diagnosis. It told me that they were standing with me. It told me that they understood I was uncomfortable and that they would do what they could to make it the least uncomfortable possible. It told me that they cared. The power of the human touch...

I was lying face down on the radiation table, again in an uncomfortable position, listening to people I couldn't see move and work around me, getting more nervous by the moment. The doctor entered the room, walked to the table and placed his hand on the back of my head as he spoke to me. Again, a small gesture; again, a huge impact. He sees me as a person. He recognizes that I'm scared. He imparts courage to me... with the simple touch of his hand.

What a powerful lesson for me.

"Then he took the children in his arms and placed his hands on their heads and blessed them." Mark 10:16 (NLT)

Thursday June 11, 2009
The "Author and Finisher" of Our Faith

Song in my head today:

"Holy, Holy, Holy is the Lord God Almighty, Who was, and is, and is to come. With all creation I sing: Praise to the King of Kings! You are my everything, and I will adore You!" ("Revelation Song," by Jennie Lee Riddle)

I have kept a journal for many years. Writing helps me to process things, and my journal has been a great tool for me to spend time with God every day. I use it to write out my prayers, to write down things that God is teaching me and things that we are still working on together. One of the best things about having a journal is to be able to look back and see how God has answered my prayers and to see His hand moving and working in my life. I don't think that is unique to my life, I believe He is moving and working in each of our lives. But my journal helps me to recognize Him in my life.

Last night I went back to the beginning of 2009 just to see what I had been praying for in my life. Here are some of my requests:

- Help me to see with Your eyes
- Help me to see the opportunities You bring into my life
- Make me an accurate reflection of You
- Convict me of Your truth
- Thank you that You are in charge of my physical body
- Help me to recognize You
- Help me to honor You in all I do
- Help me to wait on You, to rest in You
- Help me to pray without ceasing
- Help me to walk with You and to be like You
- Help me to remember that You are my God, You are in control, You are working
- Draw me deeper and closer to You
- Help me to give in to the pressure of Your hands and to be malleable
- Help me to keep trusting You in spite of anything
- Help me to understand You a little more
- Thank You that You are completing Your good plan
- Teach me, stretch me, make me, use me
- Help me to be fully committed, 100%, body and soul

Funny thing, I think God is answering my prayers!

"And I am certain that God, who began the good work within you, will continue his work until it is finally finished on the day when Christ Jesus returns." Philippians 1:6 (NLT)

"For I am the Lord, your God, who takes hold of your right hand and says to you, Do not fear, I will help you." Isaiah 41:13 (NIV)

Friday June 12, 2009

Today I sent out an email to the Community of Faith group who is traveling to Burundi, Africa on Sunday. It was just to remind them what time to be at the airport, not to forget their passports and yellow fever vaccine certificates, and to start taking their anti-malaria medicine. The last statement I made to them was this, "We believe that God hand-picked each of you to be a part of this team and we know that He is going to teach you and stretch you and use you. Rest in His hands and allow Him to do His work." And I wonder... why didn't He hand pick me? I so wanted to go on this trip, to meet the people I have been praying for, to celebrate the goodness of God toward them. I've been waiting and planning and working on this trip for a year. Why not me?

God whispers in my ear, "I have a better plan for you. I hand-picked you for something else. Wait for me."
I don't understand. But I choose to trust Him again.

Saturday June 13, 2009
Grief Comes

I wake myself up today with silent sobs. I was dreaming. I was with my daughters Sarah and Ashley. They were showing me pictures and souvenirs from their travels, pictures of all the places they went, pictures of my family having fun together, typical silly pictures of the girls together. And I start to cry, racking sobs, for the things I missed. I am grieving in my dreams. I wake up and wish I could go back to that place with my girls. I want to hold them tight. What else will I miss? The tears come again.

Sunday June 14, 2009
It's a Family Thing

One of the things I have learned about cancer is that it is not a diagnosis of one person. The cancer diagnosis affects the whole extended family and friends. When a doctor speaks the word "cancer" it feels like a punch in the stomach to the patient as well as to everyone who knows and loves that person. Cancer has a history of being a feared disease because of the difficulty in treating it effectively and in finding a cure or preventative treatment for it.

The fact that it is a "family diagnosis" has proven to be a source of great strength and comfort to me. Mark and I have received hundreds of phone calls, emails, comments, text messages, cards, letters, hugs, encouraging words, flowers, food, and gifts (it's almost like Christmas around here!). We have also felt the strength of literally thousands of people praying constantly around the globe.

My family members have made multiple trips to multiple doctor appointments with us. My family has offered to cut out my tumor themselves if they have to! My family members have collapsed on the floor in stunned silence with me. My family members have written and performed original "I Hate Cancer" songs for me despite the fact they can't play the guitar or sing!

God has blessed me with the most amazing family. I am so glad they are in this with me. I couldn't do it without them! And to all of you who feel like you need to "do something" but feel helpless, please be aware that the knowledge that you are standing with us, and that you are there should I need to call on you, is a tremendous comfort and strength for me.

"*Friends love through all kinds of weather, and families stick together in all kinds of trouble.*" Proverbs 17:17 (The Message)

Thank you for being my friends.

Update: Week one of chemo and radiation is complete with no side effects other than being tired. Week two starts tomorrow!

Monday June 15, 2009
What a Joy It Is!

Since the beginning of 2009, I have felt a very real deep love for God. I have loved Him for a long time as my God, as my Savior, as my friend, but this year it has become something even more special. I have felt "in love" with Him. It feels the same as when I first fell in love with Mark – I wanted to talk to him all the time, I wanted to spend all my time with him, I wanted to listen to his voice, I thought about him all the time, I arranged my schedule to be with him, I put him at the top of my priority list. Any of you who have been in love before know what I'm talking about. That's how I've felt in my relationship with God in 2009. It has been a very sweet time together this year.

Two days before I was diagnosed with cancer, my friend Donald Butler sent me a link to a new song he had written. He wanted my opinion on the song. He said it was a work in progress. I went to the link and listened to the song and it just made me smile – it expressed exactly what I had been feeling about my God. These are the words of the chorus:

"To live my life to know you, God, what a joy it is!

To think your thoughts, to breathe your name, what a joy it is!

To follow hard after you, God, what a joy it is!

To know your mercy is enough, what a joy it is!"

("What a Joy It Is," Donald Butler)

43

The same joy I have known all year, the same joy I felt two days before my diagnosis, is the same joy I feel today. It is truly a joy to know my God. Cancer can't take that away from me.

"And Nehemiah continued, 'Go and celebrate with a feast of rich foods and sweet drinks, and share gifts of food with people who have nothing prepared. This is a sacred day before our Lord. Don't be dejected and sad, for the joy of the Lord is your strength!'" Nehemiah 8:10 (NLT)

"The Lord is my strength and shield. I trust him with all my heart. He helps me, and my heart is filled with joy. I burst out in songs of thanksgiving." Psalm 28:7 (NLT)

My prayer is that you, too, will know what a joy it is!

P.S. I still feel that way about Mark!

Tuesday June 16, 2009
Caution! High Radiation Area!

Every day at 2:00 I go to the Radiation Treatment Center. I spend just a few minutes of my day there, but those few minutes are high impact! I am being irradiated to kill the cancer cells in my body. But I have also been given the opportunity to pray for many other people who are being treated for cancer - people I'll probably never meet, but who need my prayers nonetheless.

The sweet lady in the straw hat who always has a smile on her face radiating hope to everyone around her.

The tired old man in the wheelchair in need of strength and endurance for one more day.

The couple who had their first appointment with the radiation oncologist today, full of fear and questions.

The beautiful elderly lady on a follow-up appointment, her hair is perfect, her make-up in place. She wishes me luck.

I pray for these who God has brought into my life, if only for moments, that God would supernaturally heal them and meet their particular needs.

When I enter the radiation treatment room there is a rack of blue molds, each one representing a person being treated for cancer. On the other wall are cubbyholes with head molds in them. I am grateful that one of them doesn't belong to me. While they are radiating my body I pray for each person these molds represent. God has given me a very special assignment to change the world through prayer. I am honored to be the one He chose for the job!

"But each day the Lord pours his unfailing love upon me, and through each night I sing his songs, praying to God who gives me life." Psalm 42:8 (NLT)

"In the same way, prayer is essential in this ongoing warfare. Pray hard and long. Pray for your brothers and sisters. Keep your eyes open. Keep each other's spirits up so that no one falls behind or drops out." Ephesians 6:18 (The Message)

"Pray diligently. Stay alert, with your eyes wide open in gratitude." Colossians 4:2 (The Message)

Thursday June 18, 2009
And the Greatest of These is Love

To my dear children,

I want you to know that you have the most amazing father in the whole world! He is the best husband I could ever dream of. Ever since I have known him he has encouraged me to be who God created me to be. He always believes in me. God has used him repeatedly in my life to give me courage and strength; and He is doing that again during this time.

I know that he is incredibly stressed. I really can't imagine how he must feel, wondering if his spouse of twenty-five years will live. Wondering if our dreams of life together will really come true, or if there will be time apart, waiting for a sweet reunion. I'm sure he is thinking of the two rocking chairs, and life like our role models the O'Briens. Hoping, dreaming, wishing, praying. I can't imagine the feeling of helplessness when your loved one has to walk the path alone, wishing you could do it for them.

But in the midst of it all he has been a rock for me. He has taken on the job of all the phone calls – to family, to friends, to doctors. He shields me and protects me from things that might overwhelm me. He gathers information. He has assigned himself the job of radiation chauffeur, daily driving me for treatments. He makes fresh fruit and vegetable juice for me every morning so that my body will have the cancer-fighting nutrients it needs. He has been a sounding board for my fears, frustrations, anger, hopes, and revelation. He hasn't wavered in his faith. He is consistent in prayer and Bible study, crying out to God and trusting Him for grace whatever comes our way.

I can't be in the sun or in the chlorine of the pool during treatment because it could further damage my radiated skin. Last night as the sun fell into beautiful pinks and blues across the sky he went outside and put one of our patio chairs onto the sundeck of the pool. He told me he made a "Princess Chair" for me so that I could be in the pool with him. It brought tears to my eyes. We spent an hour in the pool, Mark all the way in, and me with my feet in, just talking and laughing together. My favorite way to spend the evening…

Your father is my hero.

"...And when we grow old
I will find two chairs
And set them close
Each sun-lit day
That you and I –
In quiet joy –
May rock the world away."
"In Our Time," by Robert Sexton

Friday June 19, 2009

There is a new song called "Can't Take Away" by Mikeschair being played on the radio recently and the chorus has been stuck in my head today:
"You can take away everything that I've been holding.
You can take away the sun.
You can take away the very air that I've been breathing.
But you can't take away my God."

I am clinging to the knowledge that nothing can separate me from my God.

Monday June 22, 2009
Sacrifice of Thanksgiving

Have you ever received a gift that you didn't ask for or want? Or maybe a gift you weren't sure that you needed? Or you weren't sure how to use it? Maybe you returned it, or exchanged it, or maybe you saved it hoping that someday it would become useful to you.

That's what cancer feels like to me. This wasn't what I asked for, not something I wanted, and not what I thought I needed. I am looking for somewhere that I can "return" it. I have decided that I don't want cancer anymore.

Craigslist, maybe?

For Sale: One adenocarcinoma. Size: 6 cm. Color: red. Condition: slightly damaged. Make an offer.

But wait...there's more! If you purchase today, we will throw in one lymph node, absolutely free!!

Don't wait! Call today!

I have always been fiercely independent, ever since I was two years old and told my mother, "I can do it myself!" I feel like that two-year-old is inside of me now, running around and screaming! I am tired of being told what I can and can't do, what I can and can't eat, what pills to take when, what time to be at what appointment. I am tired of something else or someone else (God?) controlling my life. I am angry.

I recognize that this is grief too. I am so glad that God can handle it, that He's not put off by my questions, by my anger, by my doubts. He promised to never leave me, and He hasn't.

I am reminded today that it is impossible to thank God and curse Him at the same time; that thankfulness will make me aware of His presence which overshadows all my problems.

Lord, please help me to be thankful today. Cancer IS a gift. I have been given the chance to live what I believe.

"How kind the Lord is! How good he is! So merciful, this God of ours! The Lord protects those of childlike faith; I was facing death, and then he saved me. Now I can rest again, for the Lord has been so good to me. He has saved me from death, my eyes from tears, my feet from stumbling. And so I walk in the Lord's presence as I live here on earth! ... I will offer you a sacrifice of thanksgiving and call on the name of the Lord." Psalm 116:5-9, 17 (NLT)

MEDICAL UPDATE:
Good news: Finished week two of chemo and radiation with no side effects except fatigue!
Bad news: Week three started with diarrhea...Imodium and Gatorade are my new best friends!
Good news: Imodium works!

Tuesday June 23, 2009
God is Moving

I woke up to music in my head today: "God is moving, God is moving still. You always have. You always will!"

My home office has a very tall ceiling and there are windows to let light in around the top of the room. I was sitting at my desk today and I leaned back in the chair and looked out the windows as I was thinking. I watched clouds moving quickly across the sky. They were high up in the sky. The winds were obviously blowing across the atmosphere. And then I looked at the top of the palm tree in our yard. It wasn't moving at all. It was perfectly still. It was interesting to see the two different things play out across the same sky - rushing wind, and perfect stillness - at the same time.

And then God spoke softly to my heart. Sometimes all I can see are my circumstances, my concerns, my world - the palm tree. But God is moving, He is working, He is blowing across the atmosphere. He is up to something that I can't even comprehend. How cool is it to know that God is moving still? And that gives me the freedom to rest in perfect peace.

"For as the sky soars high above earth, so the way I work surpasses the way you work, and the way I think is beyond the way you think." Isaiah 55:9 (The Message)

"How precious are your thoughts about me, O God. They cannot be numbered! I can't even count them; they outnumber the grains of sand! And when I wake up, you are still with me!" Psalm 139:17-18 (NLT)

Wednesday June 24, 2009
Help Me Live

The Shook family is a book family. All of us enjoy reading. One of our family's favorite things to do is go to Barnes & Noble and spend a couple of hours browsing through the books. We even have a room in our house named the "Great Reading Room" (named, of course, after the Great Reading Room at the University of Oklahoma Library). Naturally, after receiving a diagnosis of cancer, we began to search for and buy books about cancer - books about types of cancer, causes of cancer, treatment of cancer, living with cancer, and anything else we could find. I think we now have every book ever published about cancer. One of them is so thick that I told Mark we wouldn't finish reading it until after I had been well for years.

Out of all of those books, the one that has been the most helpful is called *Help Me Live - 20 things people with cancer want you to know* by Lori Hope. If you have a friend or family member with cancer, I strongly recommend that you read this book. Your friend or family member will be glad you did. The book, written by a former cancer patient, is intended to help the family and friends of those dealing with cancer know best how to encourage that person on their journey. It is literally a list of twenty things, plus several other lists and helpful suggestions.

Here are a few of the top twenty that resonated with me, and my comments:

- **It's OK to say or do the wrong thing**. – In fact you can just say, "I don't know what to say, but I wanted you to know that I love you and I'm praying for you."
- **I like to hear success stories, not horror stories.** – You wouldn't believe some of the stories I've heard from well-meaning people!
- **I need to forget – and laugh.** – I am so thankful for my brother Cary and my friends Teri and P.J. for always providing the humor!
- **I want compassion, not pity; comfort, not advice.** – Please stop looking at me with pity! In a moment of frustration one day I told Mark, "I am not a weak sick person!! I am fine!" I am more than my cancer diagnosis.
- **I don't know why I got cancer, and I don't want to hear your theory.** – This one is pretty self-explanatory!

Thursday June 25, 2009
Hope

I awoke today with Addison Road's song "Everything Rides On Hope Now" playing on repeat in my head. In particular I love the line that says "Everything rides on hope now. Everything rides on faith somehow. When the world has broken me down, your love sets me free."

Last weekend I met two more ladies at our church who were recently diagnosed with cancer and are fighting for their lives. The interesting thing about these women, and about everyone I've met who is battling cancer, is the hope that they express. I've heard it over and over again. I believe. I know God is in control. I trust His plan for me. And you can see it in their eyes. A sparkle, as if they know something you don't know, as if they have "insider information" – a special access to the Creator of the Universe.

I guess it takes actually facing your own mortality to realize that the things we have read about God, and the things we have said about faith really are true. And there is tremendous hope in that realization. God IS good, and everything He does is good. Because of that, we have hope for the future.

"Hope cannot be destroyed. It calls us to rise up; it whispers our name. It draws us to believe that, sometimes, wishes *do* come true." (*Hope Rising*, by Kim Meeder).

Over and over, God reaffirms this to me through the Scriptures.

"*Give thanks to God—he is good and his love never quits.*" 1 Chronicles 16:34 (*The Message*)

"*Those who live in the shelter of the Most High will find rest in the shadow of the Almighty. This I declare about the Lord: He alone is my refuge, my place of safety; he is my God, and I trust him. For he will rescue you from every trap and protect you from deadly disease. He will cover you with his feathers. He will shelter you with his wings. His faithful promises are your armor and protection.*" Psalm 91:1-4 (*NLT*)

"Everything rides on hope now…"

Friday June 26, 2009
Halfway!

I finished week three of chemo and radiation today. As of yesterday, I am halfway through my treatments! The most amazing thing is how good I feel. If you didn't know I had cancer, you wouldn't be able to tell that I am sick at all. Several friends have been bringing meals for us during the week, and I feel almost guilty for them to do so. I told Mark that maybe I should act sick or limp or something when they come to the house with food so that they will feel like they are actually bringing food to someone who needs it.

I had appointments today with both the radiation oncologist and the medical oncologist. You can see in both of their faces a look of wonder. They are surprised that I am not feeling badly. The medical oncologist keeps asking me about my medication to make sure I am taking it correctly. They can't figure out why I look and feel so well.

And I smile, because I know. I know that so many are praying for me daily. I know they are praying specifically for the destruction of cancer cells, the protection of healthy cells, and for minimal side effects. I know they are praying for strength and for peace. And I know that our God listens, that He has heard those prayers, and He has answered in a miraculous way!

"You faithfully answer our prayers with awesome deeds, O God our savior. You are the hope of everyone on earth," Psalm 65:5 (NLT)

Saturday June 27, 2009
Surrender

Research by the American Cancer Society shows that only fifty-eight percent of people with stage three rectal cancer survive five years. That sucks. And honestly, it makes me want to vomit. I don't usually think about the numbers because they freak me out. And I know the numbers don't really apply to one person, a person who is young and otherwise healthy. I honestly believe that I am part of that fifty-eight percent, that God's plan is for me to live to be old with Mark, to see my girls get married, to rock my grandchildren, to continue to go into the world and love people because that's what Jesus would do. But every once in a while, it creeps into my thoughts again. It is overwhelming. I don't want to die yet. And I panic, wondering…

Have I loved my children enough? Enough so that if I'm not here it will carry them through their life? I hope so. Because I love them so much my heart feels like it will burst inside my chest. I hope they know.

And have I taught them enough? Do they know how good God is? Do they know He will never leave them? Do they know they can trust Him completely, no matter what happens in their life? Even if their mother dies? Do they know?

I had similar thoughts the night before each of them entered kindergarten! Had I prepared them to face the world? Funny how life comes back around. And again as we left the country to be missionaries in Mexico, would my kids be OK? Every time God assured me that I could trust Him to take care of my kids. He reminds me again.

"All your children will be taught by the Lord, and great will be your children's peace." Isaiah 54:13 (NIV)

And, again, I surrender to His plan. I want to live. I don't want my children to hurt. But more than anything I want God to do what's best for them. I want God to do whatever will bring honor and glory to His name; whatever will accomplish His purpose in our lives. And I say, "Come Kingdom of God, be done will of God" in my life, and in the life of my family.

Monday June 29, 2009
Peter's Chances

Sunday morning I woke up determined to go to church. I knew three back-to-back worship services would tire me out physically, but I also knew that I needed the spiritual and emotional encouragement of being with my Community of Faith family. We have the most amazing church family!

After my mini-meltdown on Saturday night, I needed to be reminded of God's goodness and His love for me. Boy was I ever! As I was standing in the lobby of our church between services, a friend came up to me and said, "You know what the chances were that Peter could walk on water?" And then he made a big zero with his hand. This reminder stopped me in my tracks! What a profound moment for me! Zero percent chance that Peter could walk on water...but he did! Thank you God for a new perspective. Thank you for encouraging me.

"So speak encouraging words to one another. Build up hope so you'll all be together in this, no one left out, no one left behind. I know you're already doing this; just keep on doing it." 1 Thessalonians 5:11 *(The Message)*

"Let's see how inventive we can be in encouraging love and helping out, not avoiding worshiping together as some do but spurring each other on, especially as we see the big Day approaching." Hebrews 10:25 *(The Message)*

Tuesday June 30, 2009
Miracles Happen

Yesterday I called one of my dearest friends, Rose, to tell her the news. Mark and I have known Rose and her family for twenty-two years. They took us in and loved on us when we were in our first full-time ministry position. They have loved my three children as their own. They were at the hospital for the birth of both of our girls. I had avoided making this phone call for a while. These aren't phone calls I like to make.

Rose's response to my voice on the phone: "What a great surprise to talk to you!"

My thought: *Not so much, really,* knowing what I am about to tell her.

Then I told her the news, and I left her at work, heading out to show houses to clients, in tears. Great day. Thanks, Laura. She called me later and was still crying; I assured her that everything is going to be all right. And she assured me of the same thing.

Rose and her family lived through the nightmare and miracle of cancer just a couple of years ago. She called me back that night to share with me the Scripture verse she hung on to during that time:

"They do not fear bad news; they confidently trust the Lord to care for them. They are confident and fearless and can face their foes triumphantly." Psalm 112:7-8 (NLT)

Thank you, Rose, for reminding me again that our God is a God of miracles! I love you!

"Miracles fill the space that is given to them. They can be as small as a twinkle or larger than the midnight sky. However, unlike dreams, miracles come to life. They are powered by the smile of an Almighty God and profoundly change all who are touched by them. Many have said, 'Seeing is believing,' when in reality just the opposite is true: *'Believing* is seeing.'" (*Hope Rising*, by Kim Meeder)

"Faith is the confidence that what we hope for will actually happen; it gives us assurance about things we cannot see." Hebrews 11:1 (NLT)

Wednesday July 1, 2009
Typical Day

I am progressively more fatigued with each day of cancer treatment. The doctors told me that the effects would be cumulative, but I didn't want to believe them. They were right. So I spend most of my days resting, trying to do the right thing. Preserving my energy so that my body can use it to fight this disease.

Here is what my typical day looks like: Wake up. Sit on the couch. Read my Bible. Pray. Eat breakfast. Wait thirty minutes. Take my chemo pills. Wish I didn't have cancer. Sit on the couch.

Rest. Read. Think. Wish I didn't have cancer. Lay on the couch. Rest. Check email. Wish I didn't have cancer. Move to the other couch. Sit. Rest. Read. Wait. Wish I didn't have cancer. 1:30 - drive to radiation. Really wish I didn't have cancer. Come home, exhausted. Sleep on the couch. Eat dinner. Wait 30 minutes. Take my chemo pills. Wish I didn't have cancer. Lay on the couch. Rest. Watch TV. Wish I didn't have cancer. Go to bed.

Of course, interspersed in there are many trips to the bathroom dealing with the effects of cancer and cancer treatment and a thousand glasses of water.

I think I'll get rid of that couch when I'm well. I won't want to see it anymore.

So today I decide I'm not going to be a sick person. I am going to take our dog Biscuit to the groomer. It's his 13th birthday! And I'll run a couple of errands while I'm out, and pick up a few things at the grocery story. Surely I am not too fatigued to do that, right?

My stomach has been cramping all morning, but I load Biscuit and the dry cleaning into the car and head out. I park in front of PetSmart and get out of the car. By the time I walk around the car to get the dog out my stomach lets me know this was not a good idea. I jump back in the car and race over to Chik-fil-a. I crack the windows, jump out of the car, praying for the dog as I leave him in the Houston heat, and run into Chik-fil-a, straight to the restrooms. Thankfully, there is no one in there. Maybe I should have stayed home on the couch.

The dog survived the heat and we make it to PetSmart. Next on the list: the cleaners. I go to pick up a couple of things I had cleaned and the guy can't find one of them. How do you misplace a comforter? I am waiting in the cleaners feeling like I am going to pass out. I really just want to lie down on the floor at the cleaners. Thankfully there is a chair so I sit and wait.

Unfortunately, there is a mirror on the wall. I am one of those people who naturally have dark circles under my eyes. Combined with my lack of sleep last night, I realize that I look pretty bad. I look like your neighborhood zombie out running errands! I can hear it now, "Don't worry kids, it's not really a zombie. That's just our pastor's wife."

Finally he finds my comforter and I go to put everything in the car. Of course, with a big comforter it is awkward and I end up dropping my purse, upside down, in the parking lot. Everything falls out of the purse, including my emergency supply of baby wipes, and begins to roll across the parking lot. By this point, I am laughing, my stomach is cramping again, and I realize that cancer can be funny. I gather everything up, leaving the coins on the ground for some little kid to find, and head to the grocery store. I know where the bathroom is in Kroger.

I arrive home, only an hour and a half after I left and I'm so thankful to see that couch! And guess what's waiting for me? A friend brought me homemade chicken noodle soup! She'll never know how much I needed it at that exact moment. God is still here, and He is still good! I think I'll rest on the couch for a while.

"Praise the Lord, all you nations. Praise him, all you people of the earth. For he loves us with unfailing love; the faithfulness of the Lord endures forever. Praise the Lord!" Psalm 117 (NLT)

Thursday July 2, 2009
From Sarah

I finished week four of oral chemotherapy and radiation today! Two weeks to go! The side effects are still minimal and manageable.

I received this sweet message from my daughter Sarah today, definitely giving me courage to persevere.

Hey Mamba! I miss you a lot! I read your blog and it made me cry because I hadn't read it in a while.... thanks a lot!

And you have of course loved me enough and taught me enough. For example, you have taught me:

1. How models pose, because you know of course

2. Peanut butter toast and Cheetos can always make a good lunch

3. It doesn't matter if you have twelve pairs of little black heels, you can always use one more.

4. Threatening your children with throwing away their stuff if they don't pick it up doesn't work!

5. Informal gymnastics or dancing in the kitchen is perfectly normal.

6. Pralines and cream ice cream is the best one, hands down!

7. Exercising is good, but not as good as eating another piece of bread.

8. Loving your family is most important!

That's just a sampling; I'll have to write down some more later!

I love you and miss you! Tell dad heyheyhey! And that I love him too!!!

I have definitely learned more from my kids than they've ever learned from me! Family is the most important, and mine is the best!

Saturday July 4, 2009
God's Timing

God has been speaking to me lately about His timing, reminding me that his timing and my timing are two different things. Very different.

Dictionary.com defines timing as "the selecting of the best time or speed for doing something in order to achieve the desired or maximum result."

Thursday was not a good day for me. I woke up fighting. And

I wasn't fighting cancer; I was fighting God.

I don't want to take this medicine. I don't want to rest. I don't want to have radiation. I don't want to be a sick person. I don't want to have surgery. I don't want to feel fatigued. I don't want to...

I cried a lot of tears on Thursday. They came easily, and unwanted.

At the end of the day the doorbell rang. It was a sweet friend from our church bringing dinner. I had forgotten she was coming. After putting all the food on the counter she handed me a gift bag and quickly left. I walked back inside and looked at the bag. This is what it said,

"You keep track of all my sorrows. You have collected all my tears in your bottle. You have recorded each one in your book." Psalm 56:8 (NLT)

God knew exactly what I needed and He knew exactly when I needed it. Why do I so easily forget?

"He has made everything beautiful in its time." Ecclesiastes 3:11 (NIV)

God's timing was perfect this day. It will be perfect every day of my life. Lord, help me to remember.

Sunday July 5, 2009
My Rear Guard

As you know, radiation is a form of controlled burning. The tissues that are radiated end up very irritated and inflamed. I'll let you put two and two together and figure out which of my tissues are irritated and inflamed. Another side effect of radiation is itchy skin. I have a serious case of it! Sometimes it is so bad that it wakes me up in the night and I think I am going to die! The doctor gave me some cream to use and it helps a little, but not much. I have two more weeks of chemo and radiation and I have been told that the side effects could last for up to four weeks after I finish treatments. I may die of "itch"!

I was reading my Bible before I left for church this morning and I read this verse in Isaiah 52:12,

"But you will not leave in haste or go in flight; for the Lord will go before you, the God of Israel will be your rear guard." (NIV)

I laughed out loud! God is my "rear guard!" I am praying that He literally will be. God definitely has a sense of humor!

Monday July 6, 2009
Small Things

Mark and I served as missionaries in Mexico City for many years. One of my goals as a missionary was to never look like a missionary - no offense to my many missionary friends! But you know what I mean. I grew up going to church and whenever missionaries would come to visit they were always dressed differently, a little out of style, long skirts and Ked's tennis shoes. I always thought it was kind of weird until I became a missionary, then I understood. Living outside the U.S., styles are different, shopping is not always readily available, and resources are limited. And honestly, priorities change and stylish clothing drops pretty far down the list. Nevertheless, it remained one of my goals not to look like a "missionary."

I have the same goal as a cancer patient - not to look like a sick person! I don't know how long it will last, but for now, that's the goal! I dress nicely to go to radiation and doctor's appointments. I am still exercising. I have been eating while I have an appetite to keep the weight on my body in case at some point I begin to lose weight. I try to get a full night's sleep.

In spite of all that, the Sunday before last I felt horrible. I was so very tired. I thought to myself, if I look how I feel, then I look awful! Another zombie moment! The funny thing was that everyone kept telling me how I looked beautiful that day. I thought they were just being kind to me.

Later, at home, I happened to glance at my face in the mirror and I was so surprised! No sleepy eyes, no dark circles, no pale cheeks! I didn't look how I was feeling! I looked like my normal self! And I smiled. I knew this was a gift from God to me. Just a reminder that He was there, and He cared about me. He even cared about something as silly as my goal to not look like a sick person! God is good to me. Knowing His love is sweet.

Thank you, God, that you care about the things I care about because you care about me. Thank you for your kindness toward me each day. You are an amazing, awesome, good, and kind God and I love you!

"My tongue will speak of your righteousness and of your praises all day long." Psalm 35:28 (NIV)

"How priceless is your unfailing love." Psalm 36:7 (NIV)

Tuesday July 7, 2009
Free Fall

Last Sunday my father-in-law preached at our church. He has been a pastor for more than fifty years and brings such wisdom to all of us. He spoke about the fact that God compares himself to an eagle in Scripture. He painted a beautiful picture of the majesty and strength of an eagle. And then he shared this verse:

"(God is) like an eagle that stirs up its nest and hovers over its young, that spreads its wings to catch them and carries them on its pinions." Deuteronomy 32:11 (NLT)

This verse touched me so deeply that I don't think I heard anything else he said that day.

God stirs up the nest. That's certainly what He's done at the Shook house! He did it because He knew it was necessary. He knew it was for the best. He knew it would produce growth and strength. He knew it would give me wings.

It reminds me of the many times as a mother I've had to stir up the nest in the lives of my children: moving them so many times, taking them out of their culture into something different, leaving them in tears at the gate of Alexander Bain School in Mexico City, and again at Idyllwild Arts Academy, watching them say goodbye, again, to their family, to their friends, to all they knew. Stirring the nest. And then one by one moving them into the dorm, hugging them fiercely and driving away. It is incredibly difficult and painful to stir the nest.

And that's the thing that touched me. God stirs the nest. He knows it's good. But it tears His heart out just the same as it tore mine out when I had to stir the nest. God knew cancer was coming. He knew the journey would be a challenge. He knew it would be painful. And He hurts too. I was overcome with the realization of His intimate knowledge of all I am going through and the fact that He hurts with me. That's the God I have.

And the most beautiful part of the verse - God hovers over me. Even as I am falling from the nest, and struggling to take flight, He is right there hovering over me, just in case. His eye is focused on me. He is watching. And should I tire, or should I give up, should I come near to crashing to the ground, He will spread out his wings to catch me and He will carry me. What beautiful peace comes from knowing that my God is intimately involved in this with me!

A couple of years ago I went skydiving. I had always dreamed of doing it and it was amazing! The most exhilarating part was the initial jump from the plane. We were free falling at 140 miles an hour and yet it felt like we were floating. That's the picture I have now. I am in a free fall, but I have such an incredible peace and sense of beauty as I float to the ground knowing that God is hovering over me. Nothing can go wrong! His eye is on me. I can rest.

Wednesday July 8, 2009
The View from the Other Side

One of my favorite books is *The Secret Place of Strength* by Marie Chapian. It never fails to give me hope and to remind me of who God is. I don't think it's in print anymore, but if you ever come across a copy of it, you should buy it!

This is what I read from Ms. Chapian today:

"Who reaches the peaks of high mountains?

Who is able to describe for us the distant side of treacherous cliffs?

Who dares to climb higher, press farther, endure the tempest of great heights?

You can.

Will you endure the storm?

Will you engage in the climb?

The mountain waits.

Climb above the sharp stones of trial and loss;

invest in joy.

Refuse to give in to temptations and despair.

Renounce self-pity.

It imprisons you.

Your heart was meant to soar with joy.

Do not allow fear to capture your best, to paralyze your strength.

Keep climbing!
Reach the heights!
I have a mountaintop reserved just for you."

When I was first diagnosed with cancer I received a message from a woman I've never met. She and her husband had both battled cancer at the same time. They are both alive and well today. Her words stuck with me. She told me that the road would be long and the climb would be steep, but the view from the other side would be amazing when I could look back and see the work of God's hand in my life. I think that is what Ms. Chapian is talking about here too. "Who is able to describe for us the distant side of treacherous cliffs?" Only those who've made the journey. Thank you, Lord, for allowing me to make the journey. I can't wait to see the view from the other side!

"How beautiful is the person who comes over the mountains to bring good news, who announces peace and brings good news, who announces salvation and says to Jerusalem, 'Your God is King.'" Isaiah 52:7 (NCV)

Thursday July 9, 2009
Christmas in July

I only have five more days of oral chemotherapy and radiation. I am so excited, I feel like it is Christmas!

I was sitting on the couch this afternoon (as usual) going through the mail. I opened and began to read a card from a sweet lady in our church. For some reason, the kindness and love expressed in this card just really touched me today and I started to cry. I started thinking of the overwhelming love and kindness that has been demonstrated to me, to Mark, to my children, and to my parents and family during the past six weeks... and again it seemed like Christmas!

So many gifts under the tree. God's love lived out every time we turn around.

When my children were little one of my goals was to teach them to see God and to recognize His goodness and love all around them. We used to enjoy taking walks and collecting things – rocks, flowers, sticks, bugs, leaves. With each new treasure I would try to find a way to point them to God. "Isn't it amazing all the leaves that God made on that tree," or "God must be really strong to make a rock that big!" or "Wow! God is so creative to make so many different kinds of butterflies."

And today, I decided to do the same thing on my walk through cancer. "Wow! God is so good! Isn't it amazing..."

- I have had no nausea at all
- I have had no migraine headaches through this whole treatment. I always get migraines when I am physically and emotionally exhausted, but I haven't had any!
- All my blood work has remained good during treatment
- I have not had Hand Foot Syndrome, which is a common side effect of my chemotherapy drug
- I still have a good appetite and have lost very little weight
- I have kept my sense of humor
- I have had no need for pain medication
- My fatigue has been manageable
- And, I was able to go get a manicure and pedicure without excusing myself to run to the bathroom!

What special gifts from God - Christmas in July!

There is a song called "There is a God" by Sam Mizell and Tony Wood and I love the lyrics:

"There's a beauty to the dawn, a rhythm to the rain

A silence in the soul that I just can't explain

There's a breath of life I breathe, a beating in my heart

A magnificence, a scary sense of what lies past the stars

Beyond what we can see behind the mystery
I know that it could only be

There is a God; this is the proof
That all around the evidence is speaking the truth
From the center of my soul to the edge of the universe
Creation is crying out believe it or not
There is a God"

I've never been so sure of anything before, there is a God! I am
thankful for Christmas in July.

Saturday July 11, 2009
"If I Only Had a Brain…"

There are a lot of things that I am not allowed to have during my
treatment for cancer. I am already making a list of all the things
I will eat and drink and do when I am well. But of all the things
that are lost to me right now, the one thing I miss the most is my
brain! I feel like the Scarecrow in the Wizard of Oz, "If I only had
a brain…"

It's crazy what stress can do to you. I can't remember
anything. I put things down and can't find them again. I can't
remember which emails I have responded to and which ones I
haven't, or if I have written a thank you note for a particular gift
or not. If you haven't received a thank you note, it's not because I
didn't appreciate your thoughtfulness, it's because I am missing
my brain. Please forgive me.

At times, I really feel like I am a little kid, unable to think or
process information, totally dependent on Mark or the doctors
to lead me along. I see and feel it happening, but I'm unable to
do anything about it. Hopefully, before too long, I'll be able to

welcome my brain back to the real world and life will go on as before. Until then, please bear with me.

Earlier I mentioned that one of the things I was thankful for was that I hadn't developed Hand Foot Syndrome. I spoke one day too soon.

I woke up Friday morning, hopped out of bed, and my feet felt like they were burning! What an unpleasant side effect! Sometimes with certain chemotherapy drugs, mine being one of them, the medication leaks out of the capillaries into the surrounding tissues causing inflammation of the tissues and irritation of the nerves. This usually happens in the palms of the hands and the bottom of the feet, thus the name Hand Foot Syndrome. Every week when I go to the oncologist they ask about my hands and feet and look at them. I hadn't had any problems until Friday. I only have four more days of chemotherapy for now, so hopefully I will be able to finish my medication in spite of this new side effect.

Monday July 13, 2009
Room Temperature

I like hot things - hot showers, hot Jacuzzis, hot, spicy food. And I like cold things - ice water, Bluebell ice cream, air-conditioning in Houston.

Unfortunately for me, hot and cold food and drinks can cause stomach and intestinal cramping, something which I don't need any more. My stomach and intestines are cramping just fine with radiation and chemotherapy. No assistance needed. So, the doctors instructed me to only drink room temperature beverages.

I am drinking gallons of water a day to help my liver and kidneys process the strong chemicals that I am ingesting and the waste of damaged radiated tissues. Room temperature water. I can't tell you how sick I am of room temperature water. I drink it, but by the end of the day, I feel like spitting it out of my mouth. It has become repulsive to me.

The other night as I downed another glass of room temperature water before going to bed, it all became very clear to me what God was saying in Revelation 4:14-19:

"Write to Laodicea, to the Angel of the church. God's Yes, the Faithful and Accurate Witness, the First of God's creation, says: 'I know you inside and out, and find little to my liking. You're not cold, you're not hot—far better to be either cold or hot! You're stale. You're stagnant. You make me want to vomit. You brag, 'I'm rich, I've got it made, I need nothing from anyone,' oblivious that in fact you're a pitiful, blind beggar, threadbare and homeless. Here's what I want you to do: Buy your gold from me, gold that's been through the refiner's fire. Then you'll be rich. Buy your clothes from me, clothes designed in Heaven. You've gone around half-naked long enough. And buy medicine for your eyes from me so you can see, really see. The people I love, I call to account—prod and correct and guide so that they'll live at their best. Up on your feet, then! About face! Run after God!'" (The Message)

God doesn't want me to be a room temperature believer. I have to choose how I'm going to live my life. Either follow after God with everything I am, or walk away. Anything else makes Him sick.

Lord, please help me to run after you every day. Please call me to account. Prod and correct me. Guide me. I am Yours.

Tuesday July 14, 2009

Almost two years ago I was diagnosed with an under-active thyroid gland. One of the results of that diagnosis is that I gained about twelve pounds over that time frame. Hypothyroidism made it really difficult to shed the pounds. One of my prayers had been that God would help me to get back to my normal weight. Well, over the last six weeks I've lost about eight pounds, most of it during the first three days of a liquid diet during all my medical testing. Today I commented to Mark about how skinny I am now and he said, "Remember, you were praying about losing the weight. *You way over-prayed!*" This is why I married him. He always makes me laugh!

"We were filled with laughter, and we sang for joy. And the other nations said, 'What amazing things the Lord has done for them.' Yes, the Lord has done amazing things for us! What joy!" Psalm 126:2-3 (NLT)

"...for the happy heart, life is a continual feast." Proverbs 15:15 (NLT)

Wednesday July 15, 2009
Meltdown #263

Today was not such a good day. Don't get me wrong, I am still excited to be finished with my radiation treatments this week as well as chemotherapy for now. However, the reality of all that is still to come hit hard again today.

I wake up not feeling well - tired, limping on sore feet. I know I need to eat, but nothing sounds good. And then the weight of the reality of cancer hits again. The tears start to flow and I can't seem to turn them off. I'm exhausted mentally, physically, spiritually. I want to go back to bed and start over again tomorrow. Maybe I'll feel better then.

The staff at the radiation center is amazing. Nurse Rita always seems to know. I am walking out after my treatment today and she calls out to me, "Can I give you a hug?" She asks how I'm doing, and I start to cry. "I'm so emotional today," I tell her. "You know fatigue can do that to you," she says. And then, as I'm leaving, she says, "We all love you." And I know that God is still here.

Later, I am taking a much needed nap and the door bell rings. It is a delivery from a sweet friend. Mark brings the bag to me and I pull out a big teddy bear - the "Prayer Bear." The bear actually talks and one of the things it says is, "Sometimes the winds on your face are the kisses of God." And I know that He is still here.

Thank You, God, that You always know exactly what I need and when I need it!

"All I require of you is to take the next step, clinging to My hand for strength and direction... Stay on the path I have selected for you. It is truly the Path of Life." (*Jesus Calling*, by Sarah Young)

"If I have asked you to step on and up firmly - then surely have I secured your ladder." (*God Calling*, edited by A.J. Russell)

"*Remember Your promise to me; it is my only hope.*" Psalm 119:49 (*NLT*)

Thursday July 16, 2009
Gratitude

Today I had my last radiation treatment! When I was finished I got to ring the bell. The whole place broke out in cheers and clapping. It felt awesome! These are the people who have helped save my life. They have been my cheerleaders and encouragers for the past six weeks. They have educated me, listened to me, comforted me, supported me, hugged me, and blessed me with their daily kindness and caring.

I've had mixed feelings this week knowing that I would be finishing radiation and chemotherapy. These are the people who I have seen on a daily basis. These are the people who were there in the beginning as I had just begun to process the diagnosis of cancer. These are the people who told me that I could beat this.

These are the people who believed in me. What will I do without them? What a gift they have been to me.

The cool thing is that I know as I take the next step in this journey God will continue to provide exactly the people, doctors, and caregivers that I need. He is good like that.

So, thank you to my sweet friends at the radiation center, and may God continue to use you all as you care for so many who are fighting for their lives. You are awesome!

Saturday July 18, 2009
Next Steps

Now that I am finished with radiation and this round of chemotherapy, several people have asked me, "What's next?" So here is the plan:

The next four to six weeks I am to rest and allow my body to heal from the radiation treatments. The effects of chemo and radiation will last up to four weeks after my last treatment. That means I will still have the same side effects – fatigue, cramping, diarrhea, and Hand Foot Syndrome – for the next few weeks. I will see the medical oncologist in three weeks. He will be following my recovery and once he determines that my bowel is sufficiently healed, he will send me to the surgeon and we will schedule surgery. The bowel must be healed completely so that when surgery is performed it will be able to be reconnected at the surgery site without complications. Surgery is the main treatment for my cancer. All these preliminary treatments have been to prevent recurrence after the surgery. When the surgery is complete, and the pathology reports are complete, then the doctors will decide if I need further chemotherapy.

Although I will not be receiving daily treatments now, this is still a critically important time. The whole pelvic area, not just the tumor, has been radiated to hopefully kill off any micro-metastases. Every organ and tissue in the pelvic area has been affected in some way and needs to rebuild healthy tissue and heal. In order for surgery to be successful, I need to go into it with healthy organs and tissues!

We are praying for the following:

1. For my body to rebuild healthy tissue and cells in the radiation area without any scarring.

2. I have a very small open wound due to the radiation. We are praying that this wound will heal quickly without infection.

3. For my feet to heal quickly, they are very painful to walk on. In a few days the effects of the chemo on my feet should begin to diminish. We are praying that there won't be any permanent damage to the nerves in my feet

4. That I will have the discipline to rest. I am not a good rester!

All my kids are home this weekend! They have definitely lifted my spirits along with the prayers and encouragement of so many faithful friends.

Sunday July 19, 2009
My Expert

Cancer is confusing. I'm sure this can be said of any serious medical diagnosis. Suddenly you are bombarded with a wealth of information, some asked for, much unsolicited. Even the doctors have differing opinions. It can be quite a challenge to wade through it all and make decisions. Don't get me wrong. I am grateful for the specialists who have expert training in their field of knowledge and years of experience. But it is confusing to have several doctors as part of your treatment team; and many other well-meaning friends, family members, even strangers telling you what is "best" for you.

I remember one day feeling particularly overwhelmed with decisions that had to be made and thinking, "I am thankful for the specialists, but I just wish I had someone who was a specialist in *me*, someone who was an expert in Laura Shook's cancer, someone who knew my history, who knew how my body was created and functioned, someone who knew exactly what was going on with my cancer, someone who had studied *me* for years, someone who could tell me what decision to make, what step to take, someone who was an expert in *me*."

As soon as that thought passed through my brain, God whispered, "You do. I am that expert." And a flood of unbelievable joy and peace washed all over me. I can't even explain to you how it felt. I was laughing with the knowledge that God is a *Laura specialist*. He created me, He knows me inside and out. He is the one who prompted me to go to the doctor in the first place. He has watched this cancer form and grow across the years. He knew when it was time to begin treating it, and He knows exactly what I need to do each step of the way. He is even in control of all the other specialists! He is in charge of my case, not anyone else. How awesome is that! The God of the universe, my personal physician. Wow.

So no offense to any of my other doctors, they are the absolute best, but my hope rests in only One - Jehovah Rapha - the God who heals me.

"O Lord, you have examined my heart and know everything about me" Psalm 139:1 (NLT)

"You made all the delicate, inner parts of my body and knit me together in my mother's womb. Thank you for making me so wonderfully complex! Your workmanship is marvelous—how well I know it. You watched me as I was being formed in utter seclusion, as I was woven together in the dark of the womb. You saw me before I was born. *Every day of my life was recorded in your book. Every moment was laid out before a single day had passed." Psalm 139:13-16 (NLT)*

"But the person who trusts in the Lord will be blessed. The Lord will show him that he can be trusted." Jeremiah 17:7 (NCV)

"Lord, heal me, and I will truly be healed. Save me, and I will truly be saved. You are the one I praise." Jeremiah 17:14 (NCV)

Monday July 20, 2009
Mind Control

I hate to be sick to my stomach. When I was first diagnosed with cancer and began to imagine all that I would experience, I was sure that I would spend some time dealing with nausea and vomiting. That was the picture I had in my mind of chemotherapy. Thankfully, the oral chemotherapy I've had so far hasn't caused any nausea at all!

However, one of the most interesting things that happened during my radiation therapy started about four weeks into my treatments. As soon as I got in the car to ride to the radiation center I would begin to feel nauseous. This would last through my time in the waiting room, through my treatment, all the way until I got in the car to ride home. Then, suddenly, it would be gone.

It was an interesting phenomenon to experience, and very consistent. The radiation treatments did not make me sick to my stomach, the medication did not make me sick to my stomach. My *brain* made me sick to my stomach, *my thoughts*. I did not want to have radiation treatments, didn't want to be there, didn't want to have a reason to be there, didn't want to live with the side effects. Those thoughts would swirl around in my head and before I knew it I would feel nauseous.

It's amazing the power our thoughts have. And if we're not careful, they will take control and very subtly begin to affect every area of our lives. I think that's why God tells us many times in Scripture to be careful of our thoughts, to take control of them, and to direct them. My thoughts will either contribute to my healing or to my demise. And so will yours.

"For as he thinks in his heart, so is he" Proverbs 23:7 (NAS)

"We capture every thought and make it give up and obey Christ." 2 Corinthians 10:5 (NCV)

"And now, dear brothers and sisters, one final thing. Fix your thoughts on what is true, and honorable, and right, and pure, and lovely, and admirable. Think about things that are excellent and worthy of praise. Keep putting into practice all you learned and received from me—everything you heard from me and saw me doing. Then the God of peace will be with you." Philippians 4:8-9 (NLT)

Wednesday July 22, 2009
New Normal

Radiation Recovery:

Monday: Diarrhea + Imodium = All is well

Tuesday: Woke up feeling good + End up feeling fatigue = Frustration

Wednesday: Mark reminds me, "They said the effects of radiation would last 2-4 weeks." I am not good at waiting.

Thursday: Woke up feeling good + Sent Ashley to freshman orientation at University of Oklahoma = Melancholy mom

And so it goes.

I find myself continually trying to keep things normal. It sounds almost funny when I say it out loud. Nothing is normal anymore. Everything changed on May 27th. We have a new normal now. It breaks my heart that I couldn't give Ashley a "normal" summer before she left for college. At least I gave her a memorable one! I was thinking about this as I fell asleep last night, wishing I could get in a Time Machine and go back to May 26th and somehow take a different path.

But when I woke up this morning I realized that I don't want to change a single thing! I would never go back! I wouldn't trade anything for what God has given me in the last six weeks. The intimacy I feel with Him, the amazing sense of peace that has overtaken my life, the first-hand knowledge I now have of His involvement in my life, the complete trust I have in Him. These are all things that I have struggled with in the past, and now they have become a part of me in a way I couldn't even have imagined before May 27th. I would not trade where I am right now for anything in the world, not even for a "normal" life.

"…But as for me, I trust in you." Psalm 55:23 (NIV)

Thursday July 23, 2009
Dunked Again

We met with the surgeon yesterday and now I feel like I've been hit by a truck, again. I thought the meeting would make me feel good. We could get the surgery on the calendar, start making plans, etc. And there is some of that. I now know that I can take Ashley to college in August and I can go to my nephew's wedding. I'm thankful for those things. But just talking about the next steps and beyond, the length of time this is really going to endure, has shaken me up just a little. OK, maybe a lot.

The doctor talked about the surgery and what part of the colon will be removed. It is a much larger portion than I anticipated. He also talked about the fact that a large number of lymph nodes are in this area, which is very close to my tumor, which freaked me out to know. The tumor is still there! Sitting by those lymph nodes. Is it spreading? He talked about the fact that he will create a temporary ileostomy for me. I totally understand and agree with the need to have it done, but it still is the source of so many questions and anxiety about the future. He also spoke of the probable need to have chemotherapy after surgery, for up to four months! I knew this would most likely be something I would have to do, but I wasn't prepared for four months. Of course, they won't know that for sure until after the surgery and the pathology results come back.

I couldn't sleep last night. Just like when they first diagnosed the cancer. I woke up at 4:00 a.m. after a terrible few hours of restless sleep and I couldn't go back to sleep. I tried to use that time to pray for so many others who are walking this same road, feeling these same things, like they've been hit by a truck. I woke up exhausted later. My body doesn't want to move. I feel like weighted rubber. So, mentally, I am trying to readjust. All along I have been telling myself that one year out of my life is really nothing in the whole scheme of things. Lord, Help me to remember that!

I remember as a kid I would go swimming with my friends and we would always end up in "dunk fights" where we would try to dunk each other under the water. As soon as someone came up for air they would be dunked under again. Over and over. That's what this feels like. I was just coming up for air and I got pushed back under.

Lord, please give me strength for today. Give me wisdom to rest. Please heal my body and prepare it for surgery. Please ease my mind and all the spinning thoughts. Help me to walk with you today and not worry about tomorrow. Let my life be the proof of the hope found in you. Thank you!

"So don't worry about tomorrow, for tomorrow will bring its own worries. Today's trouble is enough for today." Matthew 6:34 (NLT)

Friday July 24, 2009
God Wins!

Radiation Recovery Update:

Thursday: Feeling tired + Emotionally spent = Rest on
the couch, again

Friday: Minimal fatigue + Calm stomach = Got my nails done!

Yesterday I went online to read about long-term side effects of radiation. None of them are positive things, but nothing I read was new information for me. The thing that struck me again as I was reading was the fact that I have *advanced* rectal cancer. I have ADVANCED rectal cancer. I have **ADVANCED** rectal cancer. I say it three times out loud. I am trying to get it through to my brain. This is the true situation for now. But my brain rejects it every time. "I feel fine," my brain says, "I don't even look sick. This can't be true."

Then for a split second the reality comes through. For a brief two minutes I totally come unglued. I scare the dog. Thankfully no one else is at home. Then God whispers, "I'm still here." And He wraps His peace around me one more time.

Later I check a friend's blog and this is what I read: "God wins. Every time. There is nothing beyond His knowledge or His understanding or His resources." Thank You, God, for the reminder!

God wins. Every time!

Monday July 27, 2009
"Who do you Say that I Am?"

A couple of weeks ago Mark was preaching a sermon called "Why Church?" asking the question why God established the church and why that is important to us today. One of the verses he used during that message stuck with me: "*But what about you?*" he (Jesus) *asked.* "*Who do you say I am?*" *Simon Peter answered,* "*You are the Christ, the Son of the living God.*" *Matthew 16:15-16 (NIV)*

And I wondered, if Jesus had posed that question to me, what would my answer have been? And then it hit me. Jesus *is* posing that question to me - every day. And every day I have the chance to answer Him, not only with my words, but with my life. Who do I say that Jesus is? What does my life show that I believe? Is it showing that Jesus is the Son of the living God?

This week's sermon was titled "Why Worship?" Mark talked about the fact God created us to be worshipers. We will all worship something and it's up to us to choose what the object of our worship will be. This is so important because we will be transformed into the image of what we worship. So what will I choose? Do I want my life to be a reflection of God's incredible goodness, faithfulness, majesty, and love?

And then those two thoughts came together for me. If I want my life to show what I believe, then I need to focus all my worship on Him. As I do, I will be transformed and just like Peter, my life will proclaim, "You are the Christ, the Son of the living God."

I love the lyrics to the song, "I Know You're There", by Casting Crowns. It kind of sums it all up for me:

If all I had was one last breath, I'd spend it just to sing your praise, just to say your name. If all I had was one last prayer, I'd pray it 'cause I know you're always listening. If I could live a thousand lives, bind the hands of time, I would spend every moment by your side.

If all I had was one more song to sing, I would raise a noise to make the heavens ring. If all I had was one last chance I'd take it, I would stake it all on you. If I could rise up high and catch the glance of every eye, I would make them believe what I feel inside.

If I could live a thousand lives and bind the hands of time... If I could rise up high and catch the glance of every eye...

I know you're there, I know you see me. You're the air I breath, you are the ground beneath me. I know you're there, I know you hear me. I can find you anywhere. I know you're there.

Tuesday July 28, 2009
Heart Full of Joy

This cancer journey has been filled with difficult emotional days. When those dark moments come and fear creeps in, I certainly have the thoughts that you might imagine - concern for my family, for my friends, and for my church. But honestly, some of my thoughts might come as a surprise to you. In those moments of emotional breakdown my worries might not be what you think. Here are some of my typical thoughts:

1. Oh my gosh! I might die soon and I haven't cleaned out my closet yet!
2. If I die, Mark will never find anything.
3. What about all the scrapbooks I was going to make and all the boxes of papers I have saved?
4. I can't die yet! I never finished (read "started") cross-stitching the kids' Christmas stockings!

This explains the cleaning of my refrigerator on Saturday, and the great adventure of cleaning off my desk! I better get busy. I have a lot to do!

Radiation Recovery Update:
The fatigue is gone!
My feet don't hurt anymore unless I'm on them a lot.
The small wound I had has healed!

My stomach is pretty calm most days.

Still drinking room temperature water!

"Every time I think of you, I give thanks to my God. I always pray for you, and I make my request with a heart full of joy" Philippians 1:3-4 (NLT)

Wednesday July 29, 2009
Planning Ahead

I had an appointment with the Enterostomal Therapist today. This therapist is an expert in the care of all types of stomas, ileostomies, and colostomies. The object of the appointment was for her to help me prepare for what's coming – my own personal ileostomy. I was a little nervous about going because I was afraid it might "dunk" me again.

With my nursing background, I am familiar with ileostomy care. I have taken care of patients who had them, so it was not new information for me. The therapist was very sweet. She has had an ileostomy since 1970, so, she knows what she's talking about. She knows what works, and how to care for one.

I know that they are manageable, and I know that it won't keep me from living my life, and I know that the appliances and equipment have significantly improved since I was working in the nursing field, and I know it will only be temporary. But...

When she began talking to me, it was as if she was speaking Chinese. It was all so overwhelming. Everything has happened so fast that it still doesn't seem real. I just kept smiling and nodding, thinking, "I'll go home and try to make sense of what she is telling me later."

On the drive home I decided that I'd just like to cancel everything – cancel surgery, cancel the ileostomy, *cancel cancer!* Can we do that? I'm still waiting for a response to my Craigslist ad!

Thursday July 30, 2009
Just Relax

One of the things that I have been told repeatedly over the past nine weeks: "Just go home, relax, rest, you're going to be fine. We are taking care of you."

There are a couple of strange things about that statement.

1. Really? You think I'm going to relax? I have cancer! Obviously the speaker of those statements has not personally experienced this diagnosis.

2. They tell me to relax and then slowly every form of comfort and relaxation in my life is stripped away for one reason or another – reading (I can't concentrate anymore), comfort foods (can't eat them!), hot showers (radiated skin can't handle it), swimming (radiated skin can't take the chlorine), sitting in the sun (chemotherapy prevents it), exercising (Hand Foot Syndrome won't let me), walking (Hand Foot Syndrome again).

Relax... *right*.

But the most amazing thing happened. Even as everything was stripped away I found myself totally relaxed, completely at peace. With nothing left to hang on to, nothing left to depend on, God proved Himself to be all I needed. How many times have I read that? How many times have I heard that? But now I *know* deep down inside. God IS enough. He IS all I need. He truly is El Shaddai, the all-sufficient one.

God, please help me hang on to that truth as we walk through all that lies ahead. Thank you that you are and always will be all I need.

"My grace is enough; it's all you need. My strength comes into its own in your weakness." 2 Corinthians 12:9 (The Message)

Saturday August 1, 2009
Loud and Clear

Today I was spending time reading my Bible, thinking on His word, journaling, and reading some of my devotional books. The weird thing was that every book I opened, I read essentially the same thing. God will never leave me. He will not abandon me. He watches over me continually. Nothing can separate me from his love.

"*Can a woman forget the baby she nurses? Can she feel no kindness for the child to which she gave birth? Even if she could forget her children, **I will not forget you**.*" Isaiah 49:15 (NCV)

Even as I was writing tonight my daughter Ashley came into the room and said, "Hey mom, I was reading my Bible earlier today and I read some verses and they are for you. Let me read them to you."

"*Don't be afraid, I've redeemed you. I've called your name. You're mine. When you're in over your head, **I'll be there with you**.*" Isaiah 43:1-2 (The Message)

The same message: *I'll be with you.* OK, God, I hear what you're saying. How could I miss it? You will be here. You won't leave me. I don't know why God is telling me this so strongly today, but I'm sure I'll find out!

Monday August 3, 2009
Every Mile Right Beside Us

Not long after I was diagnosed with cancer Donald called and said he wanted to bring something to me. He showed up on my doorstep with a picture of his mother along with his mother's journal. He told me that she was just an ordinary woman, but he hoped that reading her thoughts and words as she battled breast cancer would somehow bring strength, hope, and encouragement to me. I cried as he drove away from my house.

I knew that I held in my hands a priceless treasure. And even more priceless because I had been entrusted with its care. It was something irreplaceable and sacred to me.

The journal begins with the words, "Things I have read or heard that spoke to my heart or that God has said to me." All throughout the journal you see her great love for her family and her great faith in God. Even as she struggled with fears and doubts she never wavered in her belief that God is good.

A few of her thoughts stuck with me:

"To God, our journey is as important as our destination. as we seek His will and go where He sends us, God doesn't just wait for us at our next stop. He travels every mile right beside us."

"If you and I enjoyed nothing but ease and comfort, we would never learn anything very important or impressive about God. We would never learn that our God is worth serving - even when the going gets tough."

"Though my circumstances may change, I pray my faith will only grow in Jesus."

"As you have helped me to grow in the past in you, help me to continue to grow through the difficult experiences ahead. May the difficulties become a time when I can see your hand clearly."

And the one thing she wrote that I have been holding on to since the end of May:

"God has not lost control of our lives, and He wants us to trust Him when nothing makes any sense."

I like that. God has not lost control of my life. He's still God!

Donald was right. Her words have inspired, encouraged, and strengthened me. I'm so grateful he shared his mom with me!

Tuesday August 4, 2009
Good News

Mark and I went to see my medical oncologist today. They did the usual weighing, vital signs, and drawing blood, and then they put us in the examination room. The doctor came in and immediately made us laugh with his good-natured humor. We discussed my recovery and upcoming surgery and then he examined me. As weird as it might sound, I was looking forward to this examination. I finished my radiation and chemotherapy treatments two and a half weeks ago and have spent the last few days wondering if the treatments actually accomplished what we wanted them to do.

He performed the exam and then told us that the tumor had shrunk! I was so excited I nearly kissed the man! The tumor has responded to treatment! God has responded to our prayers and the prayers of so many others! The doctor also said that the surface of the tumor is now smooth indicating that it is no longer growing. This made all of us very happy. This is all good news for my prognosis and for my surgery. A smaller tumor means a higher chance of successful surgery to remove it.

"But as for me, how good it is to be near God! I have made the Sovereign Lord my shelter, and I will tell everyone about the wonderful things you do." Psalm 73:28 (NLT)

It was a beautiful day!

Wednesday August 5, 2009
Little Children, Love One Another

The band Addison Road has a new song out called "What Do I Know of Holy?" that challenges me. What DO I Know of Holy? I believe God is using this cancer journey to teach me more of what

His Holiness means. This verse from the song has been stuck in my head today:

"I guess I thought that I had figured you out
I knew all the stories and I learned to talk about
How you were mighty to save
Those were only empty words on a page
Then I caught a glimpse of who you might be
The slightest hint of you brought me down to my knees.
What do I know of You Who spoke me into motion?
Where Have I even stood by the shore along your ocean?
Are you fire? Are you fury? Are you sacred? Are you beautiful?
What do I know? What do I know of Holy?"

One of the things that God has reminded me of over the course of the past ten weeks is that I am never to judge other people. God did not create or design me to be a judge of people. I don't have the capacity to judge others. In order to be a competent judge you have to have all the information, you have to have all the details, to know the whole story. If you don't then your judgment will be compromised.

And that's the thing. I don't know the heart, mind, experience, or history of any other person well enough to judge that person. I can't know any other person completely. Only God can.

If I look at how a person dresses, or what they eat or don't eat, what they drink or don't drink, how they walk or how they talk, or any other outward idiosyncrasy that I can see, and then judge them based on those things, I have made a huge mistake. I don't know the story behind those things. There is always a story.

How different life would be if I took the time to learn the stories. The story of the angry woman pulling out of the parking lot, the story of the couple in the oncologist's waiting room, the story of the stressed out nurse, the story of the child with hollow eyes – God wants me to know their stories.

Jesus didn't tell us to "Judge one another;" He always said to "love one another." We don't need to judge, just love.

"Let me give you a new command: Love one another. In the same way I loved you, you love one another. This is how everyone will recognize that you are my disciples—when they see the love you have for each other." John 13:34-35 (The Message)

"Be devoted to one another in love. Honor one another above yourselves." Romans 12:10 (NLT)

God show me a glimpse of You today, show me what Holy is.

Thursday August 6, 2009
Attempts at "Normal"

A friend recently gave me a book entitled *Normal Is Just a Setting on Your Dryer*, by Patsy Clairmont. I guess I should have paid attention.

This week, I decide to get back to "normal" life. It's been three weeks since I finished radiation. I should be able to do some normal things now, right? I'm feeling good. My stomach is calm. My feet don't hurt.

When I saw the oncologist on Tuesday he told me that I could go back to my regular diet now, no more special precautions. So, Tuesday night we go out for Mexican food, Wednesday I add a little bit of cheese back into my diet, I happily eat fresh fruit. Thursday my body tells me I made a mistake; it is not ready for a regular diet yet. Things aren't "normal" yet.

Today I decide to start exercising again. I haven't been feeling tired. It seems like a good idea to be in good shape before surgery so that I will heal more quickly afterward. Halfway into my workout routine I realize that maybe I *am* still a cancer patient. After I finish I feel like I am going to pass out. I have to sit for an hour on the bed to recover. So much for "normal".

Then I decide to test the stay out of the sun directive. It's been almost three weeks since I finished taking the chemotherapy pills, surely it won't still cause my skin to burn more quickly. I take my book outside and sit by the pool for twenty minutes. By the time I come inside I realize that what the doctors told me is true. The effects of chemotherapy and radiation will last two to four weeks after you finish treatments. Good thing I came inside when I did!

All my attempts at getting back to "normal" failed this week. I guess "normal" really is just a setting on my dryer! I think I'll go back to resting on the couch! It is safer there!

Saturday August 8, 2009
All I Have

I woke up this morning with the thought, "Today is a gift from God. Don't let it pass you by."

Since coming face to face with my mortality, I have naturally given a lot of thought to the future (or lack of one?), but I have also begun to realize again what a gift each day is. It's really all we have. Yesterday is gone. Tomorrow isn't guaranteed. Today is all I have. And it's all you have.

So, take time today to count your blessings. Make sure your spouse knows you love him/her. Tell your kids today how much you love them and how proud you are to be their parents. Tell your friends how much you appreciate their honesty and faithfulness to you. If you love your job, tell your boss. If you appreciate your employees, let them know. If someone has encouraged you, encourage him or her back! If someone has been kind to you, pass it on. Express your gratefulness. We so often forget to say what we feel. Give. You can't keep it anyway, so give it away.

Today is a gift.

"As a result of your ministry, they will give glory to God. For your generosity to them and to all believers will prove that you are obedient to the Good News of Christ. And they will pray for you with deep affection because of the overflowing grace God has given to you. Thank God for this gift too wonderful for words." 2 Corinthians 9:13-15 (NLT)

Thursday August 12, 2009
Imagination

I am reminded again today that worry is a choice. All my life I have been a very good worrier, and over the years God has been slowly teaching me His truth in relation to worry. Or maybe He's not *teaching* me slowly; maybe I'm just *learning* slowly!

My surgery is twelve days away. As it gets closer I find myself beginning to worry. What will they find? What if the cancer is in multiple lymph nodes and not just one? What if...what if...what if...?

Imagination is a wonderful thing, but when used in the wrong way it can lead to worry. Every headache becomes a brain tumor, every gas pain is a metastasis, every muscle twinge is bone cancer.

And then I open my Bible today and read these words in Luke 12:25: "*Can all your worries add a single moment to your life?*" (NLT)

I almost laugh out loud. Oh yeah, I forgot for a second, I don't have to worry. I can choose to trust God instead. I can turn my crazy thoughts into prayers; prayers of praise and thanksgiving because my God IS the Lord God Almighty. He IS the King of Kings. He IS my everything. I really don't have anything to worry about.

Sunday August 16, 2009
Why?

One of the questions that I have been asked over the years is "Why?" "Why do bad things happen to good people?" "If I am trying to live my life for Christ then whey do bad things keep happening to me?"

This question was raised again this weekend and I began to wonder.

Maybe the problem is not why God would allow these things to happen. Maybe the problem is *my* definition of "bad." Maybe *bad* things never happen to me. Difficult things, challenging things, tough things, horrific things, tragic things, yes, but "bad" things? I don't think so.

Psalm 119:68 says this about God, *"You are good, and do only good..."* (NLT)

I'm not saying that the difficult, challenging, tough, horrific, tragic things come from God, but I am saying that He is good and everything He does is good. And if He is good, and He allowed these "bad" things into my life, then maybe, just maybe, they aren't "bad" after all. No matter how horrible they may seem according to my definition and understanding of life, the One who knows all and sees all and has all understanding of the past, present, and future, determined that this "bad" circumstance would serve a good purpose. I may never understand that in my human condition, but that's OK. I trust that He is good.

Isaiah 61 tells us that Jesus came to give us a crown of beauty instead of ashes, the oil of gladness instead of mourning, and a garment of praise instead of a spirit of despair. So whatever "bad" may happen in my life, God plans to transform it into something good.

"And we know that in all things God works for the good of those

who love him," Romans 8:28 NIV

Thank You, God, for a new perspective and for a tiny glimpse of who You are. Help me always to remember that You ARE good and everything You do is good.

Monday August 17, 2009
Wow, God!

Today I woke up back in "medical mode." I had an appointment with the surgeon and an appointment to pre-register at the hospital for my stay with them next week. I was not terribly excited about seeing the surgeon, knowing that he planned to perform a physical exam with his lovely instruments of torture.

Just as expected, he did an exam with his nice little scope. But as he was examining me he said these words, "I can't even see the tumor anymore!" I almost fell off the table! The tumor is no longer visible! Wow, God!

This doesn't change the treatment plan or surgery plan, but it does mean that the tumor responded miraculously to the radiation and chemotherapy! He said this is the very best possible scenario as far as being cured and the possibility of recurrence is concerned. They still need to do surgery since the tumor had grown through the wall and into at least one lymph node and the fat tissue around the rectum. But my chance for a full recovery is great due to the dramatic response of the tumor.

I came home and danced with Ashley, the dog and the cat; and I couldn't get the smile off my face for the rest of the day!

"The Lord keeps you from all harm and watches over your life. The Lord keeps watch over you as you come and go, both now and forever." Psalm 121:7- 8 (NLT)

Tuesday August 18, 2009
One Week Till Surgery...

Today started off with another visit with the Enterostomal
Therapist. I watched an informative video about living with an
ileostomy. All the people on the video assure me that I will be
able to enjoy all the same activities I normally do even with an
ileostomy. They made it all seem so ordinary and simple.

Then she took measurements of my body to select the
best spot for placement of the ileostomy. Her measurements
confirmed that I am short. No surprise there! She says I will want
to use a short ileostomy bag. She looked at the type of clothes
I normally wear, looked at my bone structure, other abdominal
scars, and the location of a particular abdominal muscle (I was
kind of surprised that she found an abdominal muscle at all!)
Then she took out a sharp instrument and carved a small X on my
stomach. She really should have warned me before she did this!
It's just a scratch, but it did sting! The surgeon will do his best to
place the stoma where the X is if he is able to.

She plans to visit me in the hospital and she will be available
to me when I need help or have questions about the ileostomy
and all the ileostomy gear I will be using. In short, we will be
close!

The idea of surgery is becoming more real now!

Sunday August 23, 2009
On The Road

The last couple of days have been crazy. This is probably not what
I'm supposed to do leading up to surgery, but we've had lots of
fun! We moved Ashley into her dorm on Thursday, spent time
with Sarah and her friends, and lots of time with both our girls at

Super Target, one of our favorite places!

Friday morning we hopped in the car and drove from Norman straight to the airport in Houston. We caught our flight to Los Angeles and arrived just in time for my nephew's rehearsal dinner. We were all smiles all night! I was so happy to be able to celebrate this special day with my family and many special friends!

When my surgery was scheduled they gave me a prescription for the colon prep kit and a list of instructions. I was so excited that I would be able to take Ashley to school and go to the wedding that I bought my plane ticket without reading all of the instructions. When I finally read them I realized that the colon prep for surgery was to begin *five days* before surgery, not just the day before. So, you can imagine what the last couple of days have been like.

Pre-surgery laxatives + 7 hour car ride and 3 hour plane ride = change of clothes in my bag! (Thankfully I did not have to use the spare clothes!)

Surgery is coming up in three days and I think I'm ready. Pre-surgery checklist:

1. "X" mark on belly for ileostomy – check!
2. Prescription for Halflytely filled – check!
3. Pantry stocked with Jell-O, chicken broth, and Sprite – check!
4. Bathrooms stocked with baby wipes – check!
5. New slippers for the hospital – check!

I know I'm ready to have it over with and move on to the next steps in my healing process! With the prayer support of so many hopefully I will actually be able to drink all the colon prep solution on Monday!

Monday August 24, 2009
Surgery Finally

The day before surgery:

- Sleep until 9:00 a.m. (Wow, when was the last time I did that?)
- Stay in my pajamas until noon (Because I can)
- Eat Jell-O for breakfast (Reality comes crashing through!)

I am happy to report that I survived the colon prep ordeal again! Now, I am just praying that I survive the imposed fast until surgery tomorrow afternoon!

My dad always taught me "prior planning prevents poor performance." I've done everything I can to prepare for this surgery. I've packed my bag and I'm ready to go. The only thing left to do on my list is this: Ask my friends to pray for me.

I think one of the greatest gifts that God gives us outside of our families is friendship! And over the course of my life He has blessed me with some of the best!

Each name brings back memories of shared laughter, deep conversations, whispered secrets, crazy escapades, heartaches, tears, and challenges to be all God created me to be. Each name represents a part of my heart. Each person has helped to make me who I am today, and I am grateful for that.

I am especially grateful for my friends who have been walking through this new cancer adventure with Mark and me. We couldn't do this without them. Their prayers, encouragement, laughter, and understanding have sustained us during difficult days. We are humbled by their generosity, by their goodness, by their compassion, and their protection. They have been true friends.

"The heartfelt counsel of a friend is as sweet as perfume and incense." Proverbs 27:9 (NLT)

Just as they have been carrying me through this whole adventure from day one, I know they will carry me through surgery tomorrow. These are my specific prayer requests:

- Please pray for successful surgery and the removal of any remaining cancer cells
- Please pray for no complications during or after surgery
- Please pray for quick healing of the surgery sites and no infections
- Please pray that my intestines will "wake up" quickly after anesthesia and surgery
- Please pray that I will learn and adapt quickly to the ileostomy
- Please pray that God's peace will surround my family
- Please pray that God will work through my surgeon and his team

"The Lord said, " I will go with you and give you peace." Exodus 33:14 (CEV)

Tuesday August 25, 2009
Only You and Me

Yesterday, as I prepared my intestines for surgery, I had praise music playing in the house all day. One of the songs that played was "Only You" by David Crowder. I sang it all day in my heart, and it is on my mind today.

"Take my heart, I lay it down at the feet of you who's crowned
Take my life, I'm letting go, I lift it up to you who's throned
And I will worship You Lord, only You, Lord
And I will bow down before you, only You Lord
Take my fret, take my fear, all I have I'm leaving here
Be all my hopes, be all my dreams, be all my delights, be my everything

And it's just you and me here now, only you and me here now
You should see the view when it's only you"

That's my prayer today. It's You and me, Lord. Thanks for being here with me. We arrive at the hospital at 11:00 am and surgery is scheduled for 1:00 p.m.

Wednesday August 26, 2009
Day One Post-Op

Recovery from surgery is going as expected. I slept a lot and ate ice most of the day today! I sat up in a chair twice, and I actually took a walk down the hallway tonight. I was pretty proud of myself! They brought me a dinner tray around 7:00 and guess what I had? Yes, Jell-O, again!

I have all kinds of tubes exiting my body! I have four incisions on my belly, plus the ileostomy. The doctor was able to do the surgery with a laparoscope like we were hoping, so the recovery should be easier. He was very pleased with the surgery. He looked at all my nearby organs and they all looked clean and cancer-free. We won't have any of the pathology reports back until sometime next week.

I don't have much pain and I haven't been sick to my stomach! I am sore, of course, and I have a morphine pump so I am able to medicate myself as needed for pain.

So far, so good!

Thursday August 27, 2009
Day Two Post-Op

Got gas? I do! And that is good news! My intestines have already come back to life after anesthesia and being surgically resected!

So, this morning we went to eat at our favorite restaurant, Alicia's. I had chilaquiles with rice and beans for breakfast. Oh wait, that was just a dream! But I did get a full liquid diet for all three meals today. Pudding and potato soup never tasted so good! I even had hunger pangs this afternoon!

The lab technician was here at 5:00 am, the doctor was here at 6:30 am, I had breakfast at 7:30 a.m. and met my new drill sergeant at 8:00 a.m. She was awesome! She had me up and in the shower by 9:00 am and walking the hallways at 10:30. She told me that I would have to get up and walk every two hours, and she was going to make sure I did it. She told me that I would thank her next week!

The night was short, and the day has been long. My muscles are sore, my back aches, but I am so grateful for all that God has already done!

- The ileostomy is functioning well
- I have had *no* nausea!
- The surgical drain is working well with less and clearer drainage
- My kidneys are working in high gear
- My lungs are clear
- The morphine pump works well!
- My room looks and smells like a florist shop!
- My kids, my husband, and my parents have relaxed!

I know that all these things are the result of many prayers and the compassion of a great and awesome God! I should sleep well tonight!

Friday August 28, 2009
I Recognize Your Presence

Mark and I are trusting that all the cancer was removed with the surgery on Tuesday. So, today was Day Three Cancer Free! Doesn't that sound great?

I had another good day. I spent the morning out of bed, eating, sitting, walking, and visiting with family. My muscles were looser this morning making walking somewhat easier. I'm still not going to win any races, but I'm improving each day! However, by this afternoon the muscles decided that they had had enough and my back began to cramp. I've actually had more back pain since surgery than pain at the actual surgery site! Thankfully, the doctor has ordered medication to help with this as well as a heating pad and I had a comfortable evening.

The exciting news of the day is that the doctor ordered a "regular" diet for me! I ate real food for dinner! It has been several days since I've actually eaten anything of substance so dinner was a welcome affair!

Hopefully some of my tubes will be removed tomorrow. We are shooting for a Monday discharge from the hospital.

God has graciously provided reminders of his presence since I arrived at the hospital on Tuesday. As I was on the stretcher waiting to go into surgery the anesthesiologist came to talk to me. After asking me several questions, he looked up at my face and said, "This is just a bump in the road." I was so surprised to hear those words. I wondered if maybe he was an angel? These are the exact words that I have been saying ever since I was first diagnosed with cancer – it's just a bump in the road. It made me smile, knowing that God knew this young man would speak these words to me right before I went into surgery.

After the anesthesiologist left, the surgeon came in to talk to me. He asked if I was ready, assured me he was ready, and then he said, "Would you like to pray together?" He held hands with me, Mark, and my mom and we all prayed together. Now that was a cool moment from God!

My radiologist came to visit me after surgery. He was all smiles knowing how successful my surgery was and knowing that the radiation treatments had caused the tumor to shrink to almost nothing. I told him he did a good job and he smiled and replied, "Well, I had a little help," referring to God's hand through the whole process. He said it helped to have so many people praying.

God has surrounded me with the most amazing medical team. I am so grateful for each one of them.

Sunday August 30, 2009
Home Sweet Home

The doctor came to the hospital today around 10:30 a.m. She removed the surgical drain tube (which was about two feet long!) from my belly, answered my questions, wrote me a prescription for pain medication, and wrote my discharge order! My brother and my sweet niece Sydney came and helped Mark load up all my flowers and gifts and drove them to the house for me.

It sure felt good to be home - back to my couch and my own bed! It felt good until around 4:00 p.m. when I discovered that my body is not actually digesting the pain pills that were prescribed for me.

My pain level had been slowly increasing during the afternoon until I was at the point of tears. Unfortunately, it hurts my surgery site too much to actually cry. I thought about cussing, but thankfully was able to refrain! Then I saw the problem -

undigested pills in my ileostomy bag. I hadn't actually received pain medication for hours! My sweet husband went to the pharmacy and asked them to fill the prescription with liquid medication, they called the doctor who agreed, and by 7:00 p.m. I was drifting off into a medicated stupor.

I have a follow-up appointment with the surgeon on Friday. Until that time I will be resting and taking pain medication every four hours! The pathology reports should come back sometime this week. We are praying that God will show those dissecting the surgery specimens everything they need to see so that we have an accurate report.

Again, I am so thankful for all the thoughts, cards, messages, gifts, and prayers this week. My heart is full of love.

Monday August 31, 2009
A Time to Dance

Ecclesiastes chapter 3 teaches us that there is a time for everything. Verse four says that there is *"a time to cry and a time to laugh, a time to grieve and a time to dance."* (NLT)

Get out your dancing shoes! This is a time to laugh and dance!

I received a phone call this afternoon from my surgeon. He had the pathology report back from my surgery, and these were his words to me, "They found no residual cancer cells." Let me say it again, they found NO CANCER CELLS!!!! No cancer cells. They found and removed eleven lymph nodes, which was miraculous in itself. Most often the lymph nodes are burned up by the radiation and they aren't able to check them. Of those that had been seen to be cancerous, all cancer cells were dead. All eleven nodes were cancer-free, as well as the surrounding tissues.

I was not surprised, but I was speechless. What do you say when they tell you that they can't find any more cancer cells in your body? I have no words other than praise for my God who has blessed me over and over again. We have all been praying for this exact outcome. He heard our prayers and He has answered in a miraculous way! God we praise You for who You are and what You have done. We praise You for Your faithfulness to us, Your kindness toward us, and Your mercy toward us. You are good! You never change.

Get your dancing shoes out; turn up the music, and let loose!!!

"*Sing to the Lord a new song, for he has done marvelous things*" Psalm 98:1 (NIV)

I do not know yet what this will mean as far as further treatment goes. Most often they base treatment on the initial stage of the cancer, so I could still face more chemotherapy. Also, because I am young, they have been treating my cancer aggressively to make sure that all micro-metastases have been killed and the cancer won't recur. I will have treatment answers after my next visit with the oncologist.

Wednesday September 2, 2009
Ileostomy Care 101

When I was checking out of the hospital on Sunday, the nurse read through a checklist of things to make sure I had them to take home with me.

- Prescription for pain medication
- Hospital and doctor contact information
- Pain management information
- IV and drain removed
- Going home with ileostomy

That last one made me laugh out loud, at least as much as I could laugh with a healing belly! It sounded so funny, as if it was optional! I started to say, "No wait, I've changed my mind, I don't want to take the ileostomy home." Then what would they have done?

Life with an ileostomy is different, to say the least, but it has been much easier to manage than I expected. If you are interested in human anatomy it is actually quite fascinating! The human body is an amazing creation and I have been given a peek into the normal process of human nutrition and digestion. It is incredible, really, what our bodies do on a daily basis!

I changed the whole appliance for the first time all by myself yesterday. It took me two tries to get it right, but I was pretty proud of myself! The bag has to be emptied several times a day. I feel like I am changing a baby's diaper! The bags they gave me at the hospital don't have a filter to let air escape, so it balloons up sometimes giving the appearance that I am pregnant on the right side of my body! Hopefully, I will receive the filtered bags I ordered in the mail soon. My stomach is still pretty swollen from surgery. OK, really swollen! I look like I have a basketball under my clothes! I keep reminding myself that it has only been one week, recovery takes time. But you know how good I am at waiting.

I am able to eat a normal diet now. I just have to be careful of foods that are not easily digested which could block the ileostomy. So, no nuts, no apple peels, no grape skins, low fiber for now. And also careful of foods that cause gas - I think that is self-explanatory! I have to drink more fluids than normal since my body does not have the chance to absorb fluids in the large intestine for now. I will have to be careful to make sure I get the nutrients I need that would normally be absorbed in the large intestine.

While my physical recovery is going according to schedule, emotionally I have had a tough day today. I guess maybe that is according to schedule too.

I am so tired of being the "patient." I am tired of hurting, tired of resting, tired of thinking about what I can and can't do, tired of spending so much time in the bathroom, tired of not being able to live my normal life. So tired of the focus being on "me". Lots of tears today.

And then I feel guilty. I know, intellectually, that I should feel grateful. The alternative to a temporary ileostomy would have been the spread of cancer throughout my body and ultimately an early death. So, I know that I have been blessed. I know that my cancer diagnosis and treatment have followed the best possible scenario. I know that. And I am grateful. But still...

The past three months have been so surreal. I feel like I've been in another body, on another planet. Every new piece of medical information, each new plan for treatment, every pathology report - they have all seemed so unreal. I still can't believe that I have really been living through this. This is me? I had cancer? Now what?

And knowing that I have a second surgery to endure, and possibly more chemo, it all makes me feel so tired.

I say all of that just to let you know this is reality for me. Don't worry about me. Don't try to fix it. Really, I'm fine. Emotional days are just a normal part of the process, and I certainly have mine! God's got this; and I am in His hands.

I read these words today from Sarah Young in "Jesus Calling": "Accept each day just as it comes to you. Do not waste your time and energy wishing for a different set of circumstances. Instead, trust me enough to yield to my design and purposes. Remember that nothing can separate you from my loving Presence; *you are Mine*."

"Let us hold tightly without wavering to the hope we affirm, for God can be trusted to keep his promise." Hebrews 10:23 (NLT)

I am holding on to You, God, help me to wait on You. Tomorrow will be a new day.

Thursday September 3, 2009

Today I had a goal. It was the start of something new at our church. The first Thursday of each month we will be having a time dedicated to praise and prayer, and I was determined to be there.

All day long I rested (ugh!), took my pain meds, ate, drank fluids, and kept resting. My goal was to have the strength and energy to be able to attend this service in the evening. God has done so much for me in the past three months, and even in just the past week, that I desperately wanted to be there to praise His name and tell everyone how good He is.

Actually getting dressed in something other than pajamas and making myself presentable took quite a bit of energy! I was nervous about the ileostomy – what if it leaks, what if it gurgles? I sat down at 6:40 p.m., looked up at Mark, and wondered out loud if I was doing the right thing. Maybe I should just climb back into bed.

At 6:45, with Mark's encouragement, I hopped (or slowly lowered) myself into the car and we headed to Community of Faith. We parked right by the back door, dodged the rain, and went inside. It was the most awesome feeling ever; I was home!

We were greeted with cheers, giant smiles, and gentle hugs by the worship team in the green room. I shuffled down to Mark's office and collapsed in a chair. My back was hurting, I felt winded. But I was there. I was going to praise God for His goodness with my Community of Faith family. These are the people who have prayed for me since May; the people who have cried with me and cheered me on; the people who have encouraged me with their words, their smiles, their notes, and their gifts. These people are my family.

The music started and Mark and I made our way out to the front row of chairs. My heart was full of gratitude to my God - the God who has listened and answered, the God who has been present with me every second of this journey, the God of the universe who humbles Himself to walk with me each day. There are no words really to express what I felt. With a smile on my face, I started to sing and clap my hands. Before long I was out of breath (singing requires a lot of work of the stomach muscles and mine are still recovering!) so I just stood there letting the praise of God's people wash over me. How good it is to be in the house of the Lord!

Mark welcomed the people to First Thursday and he gave me the opportunity to share with them the good pathology report we received this week, and our gratitude for their faithful prayers. Everyone was standing, clapping, and cheering. I know they love me, and I hope they see how much I love them, how much I love God, and how much He loves each one of them. He is good.

Later, Donald read from Psalm 34:1-8, the very verses I had been reading in the morning:

"I will praise the Lord at all times. I will constantly speak his praises. I will boast only in the Lord; let all who are helpless take heart. Come, let us tell of the Lord's greatness; let us exalt his name together. I prayed to the Lord, and he answered me. He freed me from all my fears. Those who look to him for help will be radiant with joy; no shadow of shame will darken their faces. In my desperation I prayed, and the Lord listened; he saved me from all my troubles. For the angel of the Lord is a guard; he surrounds and defends all who fear him. Taste and see that the Lord is good. Oh, the joys of those who take refuge in him!" (NLT)

I prayed to the Lord, and he answered me! The Lord is good! Thank you, God, for an awesome night with You and with my Community of Faith family.

Friday September 4, 2009
Follow-up

I had a follow-up appointment with the surgeon today. He said everything looks good and set me free to increase my activity level, as I am able to tolerate it. He even said I could swim!

He discussed the pathology report in detail with us. As I told you before, there were no residual live cancer cells found. They did find two lymph nodes that had dead cancer cells in them. One was one hundred percent cancerous and the other was fifty percent cancerous. He told us that would indicate that I did initially have stage three cancer as they thought. The normal course of treatment for stage three rectal cancer would indicate four months of chemotherapy following surgery. That call will be made as we meet with the oncologist next Tuesday.

The surgeon told me that if I have more chemotherapy then he would wait until it is finished before he reverses the ileostomy. He does not want to interrupt any chemotherapy treatment that I might have. If it is decided that no further chemotherapy is needed, then he will reverse the ileostomy in two months.

So, we continue to take things one day at a time. We will wait to see what the oncologist recommends next week. Please pray for wisdom as these decisions are made.

I also visited the Enterostomal Therapist again today. The adhesive of the appliance that I was using was really irritating my skin, causing a lot of itching! It was also a very long bag that hung down my leg and flopped around - not very comfortable! She applied a new appliance for me that is much more comfortable and should be less irritating to my skin. She also fitted me with a short bag! I feel much better!

Monday September 7, 2009
Lay Your Burden Down

I've had a lot of time to sit and think during the past several days as I've been resting and recovering from surgery. So, that's what I've been doing. One of the things I keep coming back to is my response to the pathology report. I was very happy that they found no residual live cancer cells in my surgical specimens. But I wasn't surprised by that report. I knew that many people had been praying for that exact outcome for many months; and I knew God was listening, and I knew God was good. So, that didn't surprise me. But two things did surprise me.

When I heard the news of the pathology report I did *not* have the sense of a burden being lifted off my shoulders. At first that surprised me, but then I realized that I didn't feel a burden being lifted because I had not been carrying the burden! Wow! It only took me forty-six years to learn not to carry around burdens that aren't mine to carry! I hope I am able to transfer this new learning to every area of my life! Wouldn't it be amazing to have this same supernatural peace in all circumstances! Lord, please help me to remember to leave all my burdens with You.

"Then Jesus said, "Come to me, all of you who are weary and carry heavy burdens, and I will give you rest. Take my yoke upon you. Let me teach you, because I am humble and gentle at heart, and you will find rest for your souls." Matthew 11:28-29 (NLT)

The second thing that surprised me was the realization that even if the pathology report had not been good, I would have been OK with that. The last three months have confirmed that my God is faithful, He is good, He is able to handle anything, and He is one hundred percent trustworthy. It doesn't matter what the circumstances are, He will walk with me through it, and I will be fine, whatever the outcome. For so many years I have prayed that I would learn to trust Him completely. Thank You, Lord. Again, please help me to incorporate this trust to every area of my life. Help me to remember who You are.

"Even when I walk through the darkest valley, I will not be afraid, for you are close beside me. Your rod and your staff protect and comfort me." Psalm 23:4 (NLT)

"But I am trusting you, O Lord, saying, 'You are my God!' My future is in your hands." Psalm 31:14-15 (NLT)

Tuesday September 8, 2009
Waiting Again

My emotions continue to be a little unstable. I don't know if it is due to the physical trauma my body has been through over the last three months, the emotional trauma of the last three months, or the fact that my ovaries were radiated and have ceased to function leading to crazy hormones and an early-onset menopause. It's probably due to a combination of all three, but whatever the case, tears come easily and I feel like an emotional wreck! I'm sure Mark would appreciate your prayers as he continues to gently support me and walk through all these changes and challenges with me!

I was crying last night as I went to sleep, just wishing that it could all be over, that cancer would cease to be the focus of my life, and that I could go back to some sort of normal existence (There's that word again! You'd think I'd learn!). Then today I got up, snuggled with the cat on the couch and pulled out my Bible, my journal, and Jesus Calling. I am always amazed at how God meets me where I am. Here are the words I read today:

"Accept each day exactly as it comes to you. By that, I mean not only the circumstances of your day but *also the condition of your body*. Your assignment is to trust me absolutely, resting in my sovereignty and faithfulness."

Exactly the words I needed to hear today. Such a perfect reminder to me that He knows where I am, He knows how I feel, He knows what's going on with my physical body, and I can trust Him.

At 1:00 p.m. we met with the oncologist. I was hoping to find out today what the next few months will hold for me, but that was not to be. We are waiting, again! I learned today that until this year the normal course of treatment for my type and stage of cancer would have been six months of IV chemotherapy following surgery. But just this year at the annual meeting of medical oncologists new research was presented. My oncologist is sending all of my reports and information to the doctor who is the head of the American Society of Clinical Oncology to get his opinion on whether I should have more chemotherapy or not. I was a little disappointed on the way home today and started crying, of course. But then I realized that this is really a good thing - getting a second opinion by the lead researcher in the field!

So, again, I will wait. Accepting each day as it comes to me, and trusting Him absolutely, resting in His sovereignty and faithfulness.

"*I'll refresh tired bodies; I'll restore tired souls.*" Jeremiah 31:25 *(The Message)*

Wednesday September 9, 2009
Remission

Before I had cancer, remission always seemed to be the initial goal for any cancer treatment. I had assumed that when a cancer patient reached remission that it must be a huge momentous occasion, that there would be some great announcement made with lights flashing and music playing. (I have an active imagination!) Well, that may be true for some cancer patients, but that's not how it happened for me.

In the course of ordinary conversation with the oncologist on Tuesday he happened to speak the words that my cancer is in remission. No one had actually spoken those words to me before, actually used the word "remission." It was surreal to hear it after three months of such intense and rapid diagnosis and treatment. I didn't hear much else that he said, my brain stopped on those words - my cancer is in remission. Who would have thought it could happen so quickly?

So, this is the big announcement, just in case you hadn't already figured it out from the pathology reports: MY CANCER IS IN REMISSION! Goal #1 accomplished!

Thursday September 10, 2009
The Twilight Zone

Thursday, 10:45 a.m., the phone rings. Caller ID says, "Private number". I have learned in the last three months that that means a doctor is calling me. The only doctor I am expecting is my oncologist. This is the call I've been waiting for, the call that will determine my life for the next several months. I pick up the phone:

"Hello."

"Dr. Campos here."

"Hi Dr. Campos, how are you?"

"Dr. Allegra says you need six months of IV chemotherapy." (The world stops spinning)

"I will email you his letter. Come see me next Tuesday and we'll discuss everything."

And my fate is sealed. Six months of IV chemotherapy treatments. Six more months of focusing on cancer. Six more months of focusing on my physical body. Six more months of fighting fatigue, fighting for "normal," fighting for life.

I hang up the phone and think this is the worst day of my life. OK, maybe that is a little bit of an exaggeration, but it sure feels like it today. I feel a huge weight on my shoulders and I struggle to let it go, struggle to remember the lesson I've learned about not carrying burdens that aren't mine to carry.

I look back at my journal entries for the past several days, this is what they say:

"Thank You that Dr. Campos is getting a second opinion as far as more chemotherapy goes. Please give these two doctors Your divine wisdom about what I'm to do. You're the only one who knows if I need it, if this will recur, and if there are still cancer cells in my body. So please guide their thoughts, show them everything they need to see, and speak through them to me."

And I let the burden go. God is in control. I choose to trust Him today.

The purpose of further chemotherapy is to kill off any micro-metastases that may have already found their way to my liver or lungs. These cancer cells are so small at this point that they are not visible with any screening method now available, so there is no way to know of their presence. Since my cancer was extremely responsive to the initial treatment, I have a really good chance of knocking out any lingering cancer cells that are looking for a place to call home. Simply put, these six months are to "kick it to the curb!" So that is the plan going forward.

As I process this new information today, Chris & Conrad's song, "Lead Me To The Cross" comes on the radio, and I feel God here with me.

"Lead me to the cross where your love poured out.
Bring me to my knees, Lord I lay me down.
Rid me of myself, I belong to you.
Lead me, lead me to your heart."

I am Yours, Lord, body and soul.

Friday September 11, 2009
Peace in the Storm

I woke up today hoping that yesterday had all been a bad dream. But it wasn't. I'm still here and I still have to have six months of IV chemotherapy. I do feel much better today, more settled with what's coming up.

After hearing the news yesterday I called my friend Debbie. Debbie and I went to high school together. She recently fought breast cancer and won. I just needed to hear her tell me that I could do this. She was such an encouragement to me, reminding me that I won't be alone, God will carry me through.

I think the hardest thing for me this week was coming face-to-face again with the fact that I am fighting *advanced* rectal cancer. Everything has been going so well, test results have been great; the response to treatment has been the best it could be. All of those things lulled me into thinking that this was easy somehow. The news this week was a stark reminder of the true nature of cancer.

I read a quote from a doctor to a patient this week about that very subject. He said this, "This is not a game. We are dealing with a potentially very deadly disease!"

But in the midst of all the grim reminders, I also saw flashes of hope.

When leaving the oncologist's office the other day we rode down in the elevator with an older gentleman. He asked how we were doing, we said we were OK, and then asked how he was doing. He responded, "Just another day in paradise!" He was happy to be alive. He told me that he had been diagnosed with cancer five times. They had initially given him less than eighteen months to live and that was ten years ago. He was going strong and obviously grateful for each new day. I knew that he had seen me in the oncologist's office and he was trying to encourage me. What a sweet man and what a testimony of hope!

I also read the following quote this week. It was not the first time I'd read it, but it was a very timely reminder for me: "Stage three rectal cancer is a curable disease." I'm holding on to that!

"With God we will gain the victory." Psalm 108:13 (NIV)

Sunday September 13, 2009

We had a nice weekend in the midst of everything else swirling around us. I am actually recovering well from surgery. I am getting stronger each day. I did five minutes on the elliptical machine the other day (it felt like five miles!) and today I actually walked the 1.3 miles around the lake!

I went to church this weekend! It was so nice to be around all my church family, to see their smiles and get their hugs! That is always an encouragement to me! I can tell my stomach muscles are healing because I could actually sing all the songs without losing my breath! Of course I came home and took a two-hour nap afterward, but that is pretty normal for a Sunday!

One of the things that was mentioned in the message this weekend, and something that we talk about all the time at Community of Faith, is the idea of making God the "boss of your life." I started thinking about that today in relation to my life right now.

What does it mean for someone to be the "boss"?
- The boss sets the values of the company
- The boss sets the goals of the company
- The boss sets the time tables for the company
- The boss decides what will be produced by the company
- The boss manages, educates, encourages, and evaluates
- The boss leads
- The boss is ultimately responsible for the outcome

And if I'm not the boss, what do I do?
- I make those values my values
- I strive to meet the goals
- I follow the boss's time schedule
- I learn, I grow, I listen, I change
- I follow
- I rest in the fact that I am not the boss

And I think that's what God wants me to remember right now. He *is* the boss. He is ultimately responsible for the outcome. All I have to do is learn, grow, listen, change, follow, and rest. He doesn't need me to be in control. I can rest in the fact that He is the boss; and in so doing, I am free to enjoy the beauty of each day, the beauty of each moment. Like five minutes on the elliptical machine, the ducks in the lake, the beautiful sunset, and walking hand in hand with my sweet husband!

Monday September 14, 2009
Family Legacy

My Grandmother was the original scrap-booker! She saved
everything! One of the things that my dad sent to me after
Grandma's funeral was some of her scrapbooks. It was really
fun to look through the books and remember fun times we
had together. Her scrapbooks include the usual things such as
pictures, newspaper clippings, plane tickets, theater programs,
and personal letters. But they also include carefully placed
birthday candles, leaves, dried flowers, small rocks, and even a
nail found in Colorado!

Flipping through one of the books I came to pictures and
newspapers clippings from Mexico and my eyes filled with tears.
My grandmother was instrumental in forming a Medical Mission
Team in her church. She was a retired nurse and she recruited
doctors and dentists to be a part of the team. Over several years
they took trips to South Texas, crossing the border during the
day to administer health care, dental care, eye care, and hair care
to the people of the small border towns of Mexico. I knew she
had done this because I had heard her stories over the years; but
I had never actually seen the pictures. Seeing them this day it
occurred to me the power we have as parents and grandparents
to leave a legacy for our children, grandchildren, and beyond.

My grandmother always prayed that one of her grandchildren
would be a Pastor or a Missionary. She told this to me one day
when I was about four years old and my immediate response was
"Not me!" Prayer is powerful, and God honored her request. Mark
and I actually served as missionaries in Mexico for a number of
years. Several of her grandchildren and great grandchildren are
involved in full-time ministry today. All of them are active in their
churches using their gifts for God's glory.

The reason I love the pictures from Mexico is because they are proof of the legacy she started and passed on to her family; physical evidence of her love of God, her love of other people, and her heart to serve. She led the way and now we continue where she left off. I wonder what my legacy will be?

"I remember your genuine faith, for you share the faith that first filled your grandmother... and your mother... And I know that same faith continues strong in you." 2 Timothy 1:5 (NLT)

Tuesday September 15, 2009
The Plan

Mark and I had an appointment with the oncologist today to discuss the plan for chemotherapy. This kind of chemotherapy is called adjuvant chemotherapy. The whole purpose is to prevent recurrence and prolong my life. Next Tuesday I will have outpatient surgery to have an IV port inserted into a vein in my chest. The following day we will begin chemotherapy.

Chemotherapy will involve three days every two weeks. The first day I will have a six-hour infusion at the oncologist's office. I will then go home with a pump infusing continuous medication over the next forty-eight hours. The second day I will have a two-hour infusion at the oncologist's office, and the third day I will go in to have the pump disconnected. Needless to say, I will get to know the staff at the oncologist's office really well!

The most common side effects of the drugs I will be taking are tingling and numbness of the hands and feet, diarrhea (the story of my life!), and Hand Foot Syndrome (the pain, redness, and peeling of the skin I had before). They do not expect me to lose my hair, although there is a slight chance that could happen. Having an ileostomy, diarrhea will be the most serious side effect for me. I already lose a lot of fluid each day so I will have to be careful that I don't get dehydrated.

They will also be monitoring my blood cell counts. If I experience a drop in white blood cells then they will add an injection of another medication that will help my bone marrow produce more white blood cells. This is a possibility for me due to the fact that I had radiation. The large bones of the pelvis that normally produce blood cells may have been compromised by the radiation inhibiting their ability to quickly reproduce blood cells. The doctor does not want to give me this injection unless the blood work proves that I need it because it can cause pain in the bones.

So, that's the plan going forward. Here are the specific things we are praying as we get ready for this new chapter in my treatment:

1. That these drugs do what they are designed to do - kill any remaining cancer cells, especially in my liver and/or lungs.
2. That the side effects will be non-existent!
3. That my bone marrow will continue to produce the white blood cells my body needs to fight infection.
4. For successful insertion of the IV port next Tuesday without complications.
5. For wisdom for the doctor and nurses as they monitor my treatments and make any necessary adjustments.
6. That I will not be bored out of my mind as I sit still for a six-hour IV infusion every other week!!

My words could never express to you how grateful I am for the continued prayers and support of my family and friends during the past four months. I feel like the luckiest girl in the world to have so many who love me and pray for me; and so many others I've never even met who have joined me in this battle.

"The Lord your God is with you, He is mighty to save. He will take

great delight in you, He will quiet you with his love, He will rejoice over you with singing." Zephaniah 3:17 (NIV)

Thursday September 17, 2009
Focus

"Keep your eyes on Jesus, who both began and finished this race we're in. Study how he did it. Because he never lost sight of where he was headed—that exhilarating finish in and with God—he could put up with anything along the way" Hebrews 12:2 (The Message)

In the days since being told I would need six months of IV chemotherapy I have struggled with the idea of more time spent focused on my health. I am not happy about it and I feel frustrated most of the time, causing me to spend even more time and energy focused on my health!

Then today I heard God say to me, "Why are you focused on your health? I want you to focus on Me." He reminded me that whatever is going on in my life, my focus is still to be on Him. That's the only way I will be able to finish the race! Yes, I have to deal with issues related to my health, but the main focus of my life is to be with Him.

The New International Version translation of Hebrews 12:2 instructs us to fix our eyes on Jesus. When I "fix" my eyes on something, by definition that means I don't take my eyes off of that thing. No matter what else may be going on around me, my focus remains on the object where my eyes are fixed. When I am "fixed" on something I think about it constantly, I talk about it constantly, I want to be around the object of my fixation, I put everything else lower on the priority list.

It's so easy to fix my eyes on cancer, but God wants me to move my focus and fix my eyes on Jesus. He's already won the race. I can learn from Him. He will show me the secrets to make it to the finish line. He will show me how to put up with anything along the way.

Today I choose to keep my eyes on Jesus.

Sunday September 20, 2009
Scared

I'm scared. There. I said it. I'm scared of IV chemotherapy. The idea of pumping massive amounts of chemicals into my body really freaks me out. I am one of those people who is never sick. I rarely even take a Tylenol. So knowing that on Wednesday I will have six different powerful drugs flowing into my bloodstream does not feel good to me.

I am also scared of all the unknowns. Will I experience side effects? Will I get sick? Will my liver and kidneys be able to process all these drugs? Will my blood cell production be able to keep up? Will I be really tired (I'm so tired of being tired!)? What will it feel like?

All these thoughts swirl around my head. And then I remember to tell myself the truth, instead of just letting these thoughts cause anxiety. I need to grab hold of each one, look at it, and compare it to the truth of Christ. And if the thought doesn't measure up to God's truth, then I need to throw it out.

Will I experience side effects?

"In the world you will have trouble; but take heart, I have overcome the world." John 16:33 (NIV)

Will I get sick?

"I will bring health and healing..." Jeremiah 33:6 (NIV)

Will my liver and kidneys be able to process all those drugs?

"Praise be to the Lord, to God our Savior, who daily bears our burdens." Psalm 68:19-20 (NIV)

Will my blood cell production be able to keep up?

"You give me a shield of victory, and your right hand sustains me..."

Psalm 18:35 (NIV)
Will I be really tired?
"The God of Israel gives power and strength to his people." Psalm 68:35 (NIV)
What will it feel like?
"My presence will go with you, and I will give you rest." Exodus 33:14 (NIV)

Please help me to continue to fix my eyes on You, Lord, and to take my every thought captive to You!

Monday September 21, 2009
Lesson from Roosevelt

Roosevelt was diagnosed with prostate cancer in 1999. Through a series of miracles, he and his wife Mary ended up in Houston in 2004 and quickly became members of Community of Faith. Roosevelt has been living with cancer for ten years. The years have been difficult, the battle has been fierce. The doctors, medicine, and science have done all they can do for Roosevelt. He spends his days at home now, resting, praying, trusting, and loving his family.

I saw Roosevelt at church one weekend not long after my own cancer diagnosis. I gave him a big hug and we sat down to talk for a few minutes. I told him that he was one of my heroes in the faith, and definitely my example of how to deal with cancer. For as long as I've known Roosevelt I have never once heard him complain. I have seen him on days when he was feeling good, and on days when I knew he was in pain and it was a struggle for him just to be at church. In spite of all that he has endured, I have only ever seen a smile on his face, a light in his eyes, and praise on his lips. I told him that day that I would be following in his footsteps and he said to me, "Just don't follow me out the door, little sister!"

Then Roosevelt said this, "God has been more than good to me. I can't shout it loud enough or say it long enough! I'll sing His praises to everyone who will listen!"

What a beautiful picture of what it means to walk in faith! Thank you, Roosevelt, for living your life in such a way that I can learn from you and follow in your footsteps. God remains faithful.

Tuesday September 22, 2009
Surgery Number Two

Today I had an IV port inserted in my chest. The surgery went well. However, I have been sick to my stomach due to the anesthesia. It is 10:00 p.m. and I am still drowsy from the medication! I am praying that it clears out of my body soon. It is important that I feel good tomorrow morning as they start chemotherapy at 9:00 a.m. I need to be able to eat a good breakfast and keep food in my stomach as they infuse the chemo drugs.

Mark and I were surrounded by God's peace today. I woke up and spent time journaling and then I pulled out my devotional book *Jesus Calling* by Sarah Young and this is what it said for September 22nd:

"Trust me and refuse to worry, for I am your strength and song. You are feeling wobbly this morning, looking at difficult times ahead, measuring them against your own strength. However, they are not today's tasks - or even tomorrow's. So leave them in the future and come home to the present, where you will find Me waiting for you. Since I am your strength, I can empower you to handle each task as it come. Because I am your song, I can give you joy as you work alongside Me."

Isn't the power and sovereignty of God amazing? He knew, before the foundation of the earth, that on September 22, 2009, I would be facing surgery and chemotherapy. And He knew that on this day I would open up the book "Jesus Calling" before I went to the hospital. So, in 2004, He had Sarah Young pen these words in the book she was writing, just for me. Exactly the words I needed to read today. I am in awe of the detailed planning of my God! And I am humbled by the fact that I am on His mind all the time!

"The Lord is my strength and my song; He has given me victory. This is my God, and I will praise him - my father's God, and I will exalt Him!" Exodus 15:2 (NLT)

Please pray for the following:
1. No more nausea and vomiting so that I am able to eat breakfast before chemotherapy in the morning.
2. Destruction of cancer cells and protection of healthy cells.
3. That I will keep my mind "fixed" on Christ and take every thought captive to Him.
4. Protection from diarrhea and dehydration.
Thank you so much for walking through this with us!

Wednesday September 23, 2009

Prayers have carried me through the night! I slept and am feeling better this morning. Please continue to pray for strength, a calm stomach, and no dehydration.

I woke up a lot during the night (I'm sure I am nervous), but every time I awoke I had praise music playing in my head - all the songs we sang at church last weekend. "You Alone Can Rescue" by Matt Redman and Jonas Myrin played over and over:

"You alone can rescue, you alone can save.

You alone can lift us from the grave.
You came down to find us, led us out of death,
To you alone belongs the highest praise!
We lift up our eyes, we lift up our eyes, you're the Giver of life.
We lift up our eyes, we lift up our eyes, you're the Giver of life!"

It was a sweet night!

Word to the Wise: When celebrating the successful changing of the ileostomy bag and appliance, always remember to close the end of the bag. Otherwise you will soon have human excrement dripping on your toes and bathroom floor! Thankfully I was not on the carpet. Lesson learned.

Wednesday September 23, 2009
Chemo Day 1

Everything went well today. I am tired, which I think is a combination of surgery yesterday and treatment today, and I am a little queasy. I spent 5 1/2 hours getting infusions today; I have a forty-eight hour infusion pump in a little bag strapped to my body. I will get a two-hour infusion at the doctor's office tomorrow, and then on the third day they will disconnect the pump and I will be done for two weeks.

We feel your prayers. Please keep it up. Please pray for no nausea, no diarrhea, no peripheral neuropathy, and emotional strength. And, of course, the destruction of any cancer cells and the protection of healthy cells. Thank you!

I'm off to sleep! Good night!

Thursday September 24, 2009
Day 2

I had trouble falling asleep Wednesday night. I was very stressed. I woke up Thursday morning with my head hurting, my back aching, my port site aching, and I was nauseous. I wished I could just skip this day. I don't want to live it. Unfortunately I have to get up and go get more chemotherapy. I don't want to do this. I am totally spent physically, emotionally, mentally, and spiritually. I cried most of the day. The tears wouldn't stop. I was sick at my stomach most of the day. I have no appetite and yet I know it is important for me to eat.

We got in the car to come home from the oncologist's office and Jeremy Camp's song "Walk By Faith" was on the radio. I am encouraged by his words, "I will walk by faith, even when I cannot see."

That's what we're doing, walking by faith. Hopefully tomorrow will be a better day.

Sunday September 27, 2009
Chemo Round One – Done!

Wow! I survived week one of IV chemotherapy! I have slowly been adjusting to my new reality and learning what I can expect in the months ahead.

I have such a new respect for everyone I have ever known who has had to live through this experience. You are all heroes and you deserve some sort of medal or something!

A few months ago, in a moment of utter frustration, I told Mark one day that "I am not a weak sick person!" Well, I stand corrected. I most definitely *am* a weak sick person!! I am not a good patient! (Can a former nurse ever really be a good patient?)

I don't like being tired and I certainly don't like being sick at my stomach! The last few days have been a little rough. I am extremely fatigued, sleeping twelve hours every night plus naps during the daylight hours. I have been sick to my stomach since Tuesday afternoon. The anti-nausea meds do work, and I finally succumbed to the fact that I just have to take them whether I want to or not. Diarrhea is a new normal, which is even more fun given the fact that I have an ileostomy!

All that said, today was a new day. I woke up without nausea and have enjoyed eating today. I am one day closer to "normal". I have ten days to enjoy before I face round two.

I can't even express how much I appreciate all the encouraging messages, texts, emails, and notes we have received from friends, family and strangers. I am especially grateful to those who have walked this path and have passed along advice and suggestions. I know that the effects of chemo tend to be cumulative, so I'm sure that I will have even more difficult weeks to come. I count on those prayers.

We are praying for these specific things:
1. That my white blood cell count stays normal so that I can fight off infections. I will have blood work done on Tuesday to see how the chemo affected my blood counts.
2. That I will be vigilant in watching my fluid output and not become dehydrated.
3. That I will have an appetite and be able to eat to maintain muscle mass.
4. That I will wait and rest and trust in God and His plan for me right now.
5. That these drugs kill any and all micro-metastases in my body.

Back to the couch!!

Monday September 28, 2009
Lifestyle Adjustment

I live by lists. I make new lists every day and I carry them around with me. I have multiple lists in my purse at any given moment. I love to accomplish something on the list and cross it off. It gives me such a sense of accomplishment; and now, those lists actually serve as my brain!

Several years ago Mark and I lived in Mexico City. This move was a major lifestyle adjustment for me. The city is huge and congested. Traffic is a nightmare. Traffic laws are even more of a nightmare. The pace of living is very different from how it is in Houston.

Of course I continued with my listing habit and would make my "To Do" list for each day, and each new day would be an exercise in complete frustration. I would have ten things that I needed to accomplish that day, I would spend hours out and about in the city trying to accomplish those things, and come home totally exhausted having crossed absolutely nothing off the list! Talk about a learning experience!

God used that time in my life to teach me to relax, to learn to enjoy the beauty of each new day, the beauty of a new culture and people, and to enjoy the small moments and victories. I learned to make a "To Do" list with only one thing on the list and if I accomplished one thing each day I considered that a good day.

Now I find myself in that same place again. God is reminding me to slow down, appreciate the beauty of each new day, and quit judging my life by how many things I can cross off the list. So, here was my list for today:

1. Take a shower
2. Wash the dishes
3. Change the ileostomy bag

Wow, my life has changed in the last four months! And that's a good thing!

"Come and see what our God has done, what awesome miracles he performs for people!" Psalm 66:5 (NLT)

Tuesday September 29, 2009
Miracles Again

I feel like I won the lottery today! Prayers have been answered, as always, by a very gracious God.

I saw the oncologist today to see how my first chemotherapy treatment affected my blood cells. He was concerned that they may have dropped too low due to the previous radiation to my pelvis and possible damage to the bone marrow in my pelvic bones. I know that many of you have been praying specifically for my blood counts, and the news was good. While the numbers did drop, they are still within the normal range, which means that, for this treatment cycle at least, I do not have to add another injection to my chemo regimen. I am very happy, very proud of my bone marrow, very thankful for your prayers, and very grateful for God's small mercies.

"Then call on me when you are in trouble, and I will rescue you and you will give me glory." Psalm 50:15 (NLT)

Lord, today we give You glory!

Wednesday September 30, 2009
Leaning

The last week has been another of those times when God keeps repeating something to me in different ways. Could that mean I'm not listening well? The key word this time has been "lean."

*"Trust in the Lord with all your heart and **lean** not on your own understanding; in all your ways acknowledge Him and He will make your paths straight." Proverbs 3:5-6 (NIV)*

That old hymn "Leaning on the Everlasting Arms" has been playing on repeat in my head all week. Then I received a sweet card in the mail with the picture of two little girls, one leaning on the back of the other's shoulder. The card said this, "If you need to lean awhile, I'm here."

And Mark brought me a gift on my first day of chemotherapy this week. It came in a beautiful package with a big purple bow. I opened the package and found a gorgeous Lladro porcelain figurine of a girl resting and leaning. Mark said, "I saw this and I had to buy it for you. It's you, leaning on the Lord."

Sometimes I am a little thickheaded, but I am starting to see a trend here. God wants me to understand what it means to "lean," He wants me to recognize the benefits of leaning, and He wants me to practice doing so. He also wants me to know when and where to lean and when and where to "lean not".

Just for fun I looked up the definition of the word lean and here is what the Webster's Dictionary says:

lean [leen] *verb*
To rest against or on something for support
To press against
To incline the weight of the body
To depend or rely for assistance

If you think about the times in our lives when we lean it is when we are injured, broken, weak, sick, unable to carry our own weight; and then we lean - on crutches, on canes, on other people.

But I see God's Word here telling me to lean on Him as an ordinary practice of my day. He wants me to lean daily, constantly, continuously on Him. My human condition, whether I recognize it or not, is one of brokenness and weakness. If I'm not leaning on Him, I will never be able to live the life He has planned for me.

So my new paraphrase of the verses from Proverbs goes like this:

"Laura, rest against the Lord daily, constantly, continuously; and do not rely for assistance on yourself; in all your ways press against Him and He will accomplish His good plans for you."

I'm going to practice leaning today.

Sunday October 4, 2009
Thanks, Mom and Dad!

A sweet friend emailed me the other day with some questions. She was wondering how she might respond if she were in my situation, wondering how she would handle the spiritual side of the struggle and wondering how it's been for me.

I think we always wonder how we would respond when faced with a difficult situation like cancer. Hoping that we would be strong warriors of faith, but afraid that maybe we wouldn't. All I know is that from the moment the doctor said, "You have cancer" I had a supernatural peace just flood over me, like everything was going to be OK. Not easy, not fun, maybe not even turning out like we would hope; but that it was going to be OK because God is here. That peace hasn't left me. Certainly I have had many moments of crying, screaming, grief, deep fear, anguish for my kids and my husband; but every time He meets me there and scoops me up and says let's just take the next step.

For some reason I've never even thought "Why me?" I have had such a profound sense of His presence, like never before in my life, that it's been awesome just to sit back and watch as

He has orchestrated every little detail, even down to having my radiation nurse walk into the hospital at the exact same time I was walking out from day surgery last week. She has been one of my cheerleaders from the beginning; and I just had to smile when I saw her, knowing that God had her there at that moment just for me.

The week of the first IV treatment was rough. I cried all day about everything, good things and bad things, I couldn't stop. I told Mark that I felt like I'd lost my testimony, like I wasn't really trusting God. But he just encouraged me and told me to keep going. There are days I feel like I can't do this anymore, and I certainly don't want to, but then I see what He's doing - in my life, in our church, through my story - and I know that it's Him, He's going to carry me through, whatever that means.

I have found that it is very much a mental battle for me now. Fighting to keep my focus fixed on Jesus and on His word and His truth no matter what. That is definitely work for me. I was watching a show on television the other night and one of the characters had been battling cancer. In that episode her husband screamed the line, "What am I scared of? I'm scared of everything!" And I thought to myself, "That's it!" When I don't keep my focus on Jesus, I'm scared of everything. But when it is laser focused on Him, everything is OK. Maintaining focus is my daily work.

My parents have always remained calm with a positive attitude no matter the circumstances in their lives. There were times I wondered, "How can they be so calm? Can't they see what's going on here?" Now I know. They saw what was really going on. God was in control; and they chose to trust and have peace. Thanks, Mom and Dad, for showing me how to walk by faith.

"The Lord stands at your right hand to protect you." Psalm 110:5 (NLT)

Monday October 5, 2009
The Back Room

Last week I had a follow-up appointment with the colorectal surgeon. Now, don't get me wrong, I absolutely love my surgeon and I would recommend him without reservation to anyone who is looking for a colorectal surgeon, but I am never too excited to go see him at his office.

My first clue should have been when his nurse said to me, "We're going to put you in the back room." It always makes me laugh when I walk into the room and there is a speculum on the counter draped with a rubber glove. It all looks innocent enough, but I have some experience in these rooms and I have a pretty good idea of what is in store for me.

The doctor comes in with his new fellow – a doctor who is pursuing specialized training in colorectal surgery. I fully support medical education, but I think to myself, "Just one more person who gets to know me in a very personal way!" He checks out my abdominal incisions. Everything has healed well. Then he sweetly asks, "Is it OK if I check the internal surgical site?" How do you honestly answer that question? I think to myself, "NO! IT IS NOT OK!" But when I open my mouth I hear myself say, "Of course, please do whatever you need to do."

Thankfully, all the news is good. My rectum (yes, I said the word, rectum) is connected at the surgical site and healing well. There should be no trouble for these six months until we are able to put the whole system back in working order.

Again, I am so grateful for my surgeon, for his training, his knowledge, his skill, his desire to train other surgeons, and his genuine compassion toward me and my family. I am very blessed.

Tuesday morning at 9:00 a.m. I will begin my second round of chemotherapy. We are hoping that most of the nausea last time was due to a combination of surgery, anesthesia, and chemotherapy all in one week; and that this time I will not be so sick to my stomach.

We continue to pray for the following:

- No nausea
- No drop in blood cell production
- No peripheral neuropathy
- No diarrhea or dehydration
- That my liver and kidneys will be able to process all these chemicals efficiently
- Destruction of any cancer cells and protection of healthy cells

Tuesday October 6, 2009
Change of Plans

I get up early, eat a good breakfast, change the whole ileostomy apparatus (knowing I won't feel good for the next couple of days), pack my stuff to spend the day at the doctor's office, and head out the door. I'm feeling good, ready to get round two of chemotherapy done and be one step closer to the end of treatment.

On the way Mark and I are discussing his message for the church this weekend and we start talking about the things we are struggling with and the things that God has been teaching us in the last few months. I tell him that God has been teaching me so many things but that the two things I keep coming back around to are 1. Giving up control of my calendar and my life, and 2. Controlling my thinking.

I have such a drive to be in control of everything in my life. I tend to think that I can do everything myself. I especially love to make plans, organize my calendar, and keep everything scheduled.

Well, that part of my life has been totally blown out in the last four months! I am obviously not in control of anything. Still I find myself trying to plan and work it all out, only to be reminded every time that I am not in control of things right now.

I have a very melancholy personality and often in my life I have battled negative thinking. At times this negative thinking leads me to believe things that aren't true and act in ways that are not productive. I have found over the course of these last four months that my thought life is critical, and God wants me to learn to think and live in the truth, to keep my thoughts focused on Him and on His Word. This is a daily challenge.

These are the things that Mark and I discuss on the way to the doctor's office today. We arrive at 9:00, wait for almost an hour to be called back. I get my blood drawn and then go make myself comfortable in the infusion room. We wait longer to get my blood results back, and in the meantime, the nurse hooks up the IV line and flushes my port. We're all ready to start infusing six hours of chemicals.

Then the nurse returns and lets me know that, unfortunately, my white blood cell count did not come back up high enough to be able to receive chemotherapy today. The doctor says I will have to wait until next week. I stare at her in disbelief as I hear my plans come crashing down once again. My first thought is that this means the treatments are going to be pushed back, lasting at least until the end of March now. I am in tears. I am so frustrated. God, I had my plans!

We get in the car to leave and the negative thinking begins. What did I do wrong? Did I not eat right? Did I not rest enough? I should have been able to prevent this. More tears.

And then the laughter comes. God must have been smiling as we drove to the doctor's office this morning, listening to our discussion and knowing what was going to happen to me today.

OK, I hear You again. You are God; You are in control. I can let go and relax knowing You have it all planned out. And I will toss out the negative thoughts and hold on to Your truth. Thank You for one more chance to see who You are.

So, the plan as of today (and we all know that can change at any given moment!) is that I will receive round two of chemo in one week. The doctor will monitor my white blood cells after that treatment, hoping that they will rebound faster than they did with the first treatment. If they don't, then most likely they will add the injection of bone marrow boosting drugs to the following treatments to increase my body's production of blood cells.

The good news is I get another week to feel good! I will be avoiding crowds in an effort to keep from getting sick as my immune system works to increase my white blood cell production.

I will be practicing living "out of control" this week and the art of taking every thought captive to Christ, again!

Wednesday October 7, 2009
And This is Love

Your love for one another will prove to the world that you are my disciples." John 13:35 (NLT)

You know you are loved when...
- A friend makes you homemade ginger bread to help combat nausea
- A friend sends you a box of Godiva chocolates
- A friend surprises you (almost) with pots of fall flowers on your front porch
- A friend makes you homemade biscotti to eat when nothing else will stay down
- A friend gives you new pajama pants and slippers

- A friend sends you beautiful photos of nature every week to remind you of God's beauty
- A friend brings you a bag of crossword puzzles and magazines to keep busy during long days of chemotherapy infusion
- A friend comes all the way from Mexico to see you
- A friend listens and lets you cry
- A friend spends a day fasting and praying for your healing
- A group of friends gather around, lay their hands on you, and pray for your healing
- A friend emails just to remind you that six months isn't that long and you can do it
- Your husband still calls you his "smokin' hot wife"

"But if we love one another, God dwells deeply within us, and his love becomes complete in us – perfect love!" 1 John 4:11 *(The Message)*

Sunday October 11, 2009
Our Hope

When I was first diagnosed with cancer I found myself having very vivid dreams at night as my brain was processing all the information being thrown at it so suddenly. In the last few days, those vivid dreams are back; or at least I am aware of them right now. For several nights in a row I have dreamed that I am preparing my family for my death in some way. I guess my brain is now beginning to process some of the fears I've felt along the way. It is weird to wake up and start the day after dreaming of your impending death!

In one of the more interesting dreams I was actually helping prepare a lady to go on a date with Mark. She wanted my advice on what to wear and what to talk about. I calmly gave her my advice and then sent them off on their date, as if I were their mother or something. In one dream I kicked Mark in the stomach. I'm not sure why (maybe because he had gone on that date?), but I actually physically kicked my leg out while I was sleeping and woke myself up.

Those may have been dreams, but the reality of death isn't. It's on the mind of every person who has faced a cancer diagnosis. I review my Last Will and Testament. I let family members and doctors know where my Living Will and Medical Power of Attorney are located. I keep a list of songs in my notebook I would like to have sung at my funeral. I wonder what pictures will be displayed for those who gather to mourn my loss? I make sure Mark knows I want a closed casket; such surreal conversations.

Death has become a part of life.

I read these words in the book of Revelation:

"I heard a loud shout from the throne, saying, 'Look, God's home is now among his people! He will live with them, and they will be his people. God himself will be with them. He will wipe every tear from their eyes, and there will be no more death or sorrow or crying or pain. All these things are gone forever.' And the one sitting on the throne said, 'Look, I am making everything new!' And then he said to me, 'Write this down, for what I tell you is trustworthy and true.'" Revelation 21:3-5 (NLT)

This is our hope. I am ready.

Monday October 12, 2009
The Barter System

My son David lives with his wife Sydneyann in Los Angeles. They are very active in their local community of Silver Lake, leading out in an effort to connect with their neighbors and the local businesses. Not too long ago David called and told me that he had decided to talk to the local hair salon and see if he could barter for a haircut. I laughed out loud, but David was serious! It's not cheap to live in Southern California, so he thought this would be a good way to save some money. He would offer them something he had in exchange for a haircut.

So, David emailed the local salon and offered to write them a poem in exchange for a haircut. They could keep the poem and display it on their wall, and he told them that one day when he was a famous poet it would be worth something. Much to my surprise, the owner of the hair salon liked the idea of the barter and agreed. David got his hair cut for free, and he is now the Poet Laureate of The Hive Hair Shop in Silver Lake! This was the beginning of a great relationship between David, Sydneyann, the owners of the Hive, and many of the people in their neighborhood. The barter system, alive and well in Silver Lake!

I am finding that the barter system is alive and well in my life as well. My cancer treatment has seemed something like a barter system to me:

"Give us six weeks of radiation and we'll give you diarrhea."

"Give us ten inches of your rectum and colon and we'll give you an ileostomy."

"Give us six months of your life and we'll give you six years."

I feel somehow something went wrong with my barter system. Maybe I should be writing poems.

Then I remember the real trades that have been made in the last four months:

"Give me your trust and I will walk with you daily."

"Give me your fears and I will give you my peace."

"Give up control and I will write your story."

"Give me your life and I will give you Mine."

God has given me a good deal!

Tuesday October 13, 2009
Frustration

Just another frustrating day. My blood count was even lower today than last week, so no treatment again. This is not unheard of, but the doctor had expected that it would bounce back up more quickly since I am young. Apparently the combination of the first chemotherapy treatment and the radiation treatments I received back in June and July had a big impact on my body. So, we are waiting again. I will see the doctor next week and we will check the blood counts again. He is hoping that I will be able to receive my chemo treatment then. But if the numbers haven't increased then he will give me a series of daily shots that will help boost blood cell production so that they will be able to give me the treatment. Each treatment going forward will be followed by an injection that will help keep my blood cell production where it needs to be between treatments. At least that's my understanding of the plans.

The nurse said today that it is completely out of our control. My body will eventually replace the blood cells; we just have to wait. When she said those words, "it is completely out of our control," I just had to laugh. If I've learned one thing through this whole experience, that's it. No truer words have been spoken.

Between now and next Monday I will have to continue to protect myself from exposure to infections since my body has very few resources to defend itself right now. More couch time for me.

Mark and I came home from the doctor's office very frustrated and disappointed. It is exhausting to get emotionally geared up to go have chemotherapy and then not actually receive it. We came home, cried, fussed at each other out of frustration, and then collapsed in exhaustion. It's amazing what a good nap can do for the spirit!

I called the oncologist this afternoon to voice my concern about the delay in treatment, and in his cute Peruvian accent he said to me, "Don't worry. You are going to be fine. You are OK. Don't worry. Don't worry." So I am choosing not to worry.

I read these words the other day in *Jesus Calling* and they have stuck with me:

"Trust me enough to let things happen without striving to predict or control them... When you project yourself into the future rehearsing what you will do or say, you are seeking to be self-sufficient: to be adequate without My help. This is a subtle sin - so common that it usually slips by unnoticed."

Lord, please help me not to be self-sufficient but to recognize that everything I need is found in You. And with that recognition, help me to wait for You and rely *on You today.*

"I pray to God—my life a prayer— and wait for what he'll say and do. My life's on the line before God, my Lord, waiting and watching till morning, waiting and watching till morning." Psalm 130:5-6 (The Message)

"The Lord's delight is in those who fear Him, those who put their hope in his unfailing love." Psalm 147:11 (NLT)

Wednesday October 14, 2009
Every Good and Perfect Gift

Several years ago theologian John Piper was diagnosed with prostate cancer. He wrote an article the night before he had surgery entitled "Don't Waste Your Cancer." In the article Piper says, "You will waste your cancer if you believe it is a curse and not a gift." This is something that God showed me early in this journey, but it was good to be reminded today.

With Piper's thoughts in my head I sat down to read my Bible, journal, and pray. Without really realizing it, my writing took on a life of it's own and suddenly became a "Thank You" note to God:

Thank You for cancer.

Thank You for what you are doing in my life, and in my family's life, and in my church.

Thank You for the beauty I've seen – in the human body, in people, in Your church, and in You.

Thank You for the lessons I am learning.

Thank You for the relationship with You that continues to grow.

Thank You for the new relationships and renewed relationships I am developing with family and friends.

Thank You for the compassion for others who are hurting that You have given me.

Thank You for the release of the need to judge people that I have experienced.

Thank You for the strength You are forming in me.

Thank You for an even deeper and stronger relationship with Mark.

Thank You for the freedom and peace that I feel.

Thank You for the freedom from "doing".

Thank You for a life out of my control.

Thank You for time to spend with You – to think, to question, to pray, to meditate.

Thank You for a new understanding that I never had before.

Thank You for the glimpses of Your goodness.

Thank You for the life I've found in Your words.

Thank You for Your presence.

Thank You for the deep knowing – the unshakeable knowledge of the truth of You.

Thank You. Cancer *is* a gift.

"So, my very dear friends, don't get thrown off course. Every desirable and beneficial gift comes out of heaven. The gifts are rivers of light cascading down from the Father of Light. There is nothing deceitful in God, nothing two-faced, nothing fickle. He brought us to life using the true Word, showing us off as the crown of all his creatures." James 1:16-18 (The Message)

"So, what do you think? With God on our side like this, how can we lose? If God didn't hesitate to put everything on the line for us, embracing our condition and exposing himself to the worst by sending his own Son, is there anything else he wouldn't gladly and freely do for us?" Romans 8:31-32 (The Message)

Sunday October 18, 2009
My Hiding Place

Last week, as the doctor told me my white blood cells were practically non-existent, he told me that I need to be very careful. Right now I have very little ability to fight off infection. I was told to stay away from people, to stay out of crowds, to be careful of eating raw fruits or vegetables, and to wash my hands – a lot!

I have been very careful to follow their advice and so far I am doing well. The only catch is that Mark and I had already planned to start a new message series on relationships at the church this weekend and we were planning to speak together. What was it the doctor said about people and crowds?

In order to avoid all hugging, hand-shaking, coughing, sneezing, and germ-infected children, I entered the building through the back door, went straight to Mark's office without talking or touching anyone, and sat alone, waiting, until the time came in the services for the message to be shared. Then I entered the stage from the back, Mark and I shared what God had given us to share, and I left the same way I'd come in. It feels really weird not to be hugging anyone and not to be able to see and talk to everyone. Hopefully this issue will be resolved soon and I will be back out there with the people.

In spite of the fact that I was alone, I had the most amazing experience in worship today! The band started playing the song "I Will Exalt You" by Hillsong and I stepped through the door at the back of the stage waiting to join Mark on stage for the message. Standing in that spot feels kind of like you are in a closet. It's a small space, the walls are black and it was dark. The music coming through the monitors on the stage was bouncing off the back of the stage and made for an incredible decibel level where I was waiting. Then I started listening to the words of the song, and I started singing out to my God.

"I will exalt You
I will exalt You
I will exalt You
You are my God"
And God whispered in my ear, "I'm right here with you." Instantly I felt His presence surround me.

I started thinking about being at home these last couple of weeks in a form of quarantine, and then we sang these words:
"My hiding place
My safe refuge
My treasure Lord You are"
And it hit me that He *is* my safe refuge, He has been protecting me as my blood counts have been so low. He has been my hiding place these weeks. I continued to sing,
"My friend and King
Anointed One
Most Holy"
As I was praising Him, proclaiming His Holiness, I said to Him, "You are everything to me."

And then I heard God whisper back, "YOU are everything to Me."

In that instant I understood like never before that I am His daughter, that I am everything to Him, just like my children are to me. Tears clouded my eyes, and unspeakable joy filled my heart and I shouted out to Him,

"I will exalt You

I will exalt You

I will exalt You

You are my God"

And then we sang the last verse:

"Because You're with me

Because You're with me

Because You're with me

I will not fear"

What a timely reminder to me during these days! He will be with me, just like He was today. He is my refuge. He is my hiding place. He is Holy and worthy of my praise. I am His.

Monday October 19, 2009
Chemo Round Two

Prayers have been answered! I had an appointment with the oncologist today. Last week they told me to be ready to stay and receive my chemo treatment if my white blood cell count had come up to a safe level. I brought my chemo bag with me, full of fun things to read and do as well as snacks to ward off nausea. But after my experience the last two times I tried to start round two, I just left the bag in the car fully expecting the cell count to still be low.

My doctor came in the room with a big smile and told me that the count had gone up from 2.0 to 3.5, which was now a safe level to receive chemo. They sent me back to the infusion room to get started today. I was so excited to hear that my blood count had recovered that I was happy to get chemo. How weird is that – feeling happy to get chemo?

Why am I still surprised when God answers our prayers? I should have been expecting it.

David, Sydneyann, and her mother came to sit with me for a while today. David and I played Scrabble. I lost, of course! If only there were a word that had five Is in it!

Tonight, I am very tired, I can feel the irritated nerves in my throat, but otherwise I feel pretty good. I was able to eat; my stomach is calm. So far, so good.

It is exciting to see that God answered our specific prayers. Today we are praying for minimal and manageable side effects over the next few days.

Wednesday October 21, 2009
Two Down, Ten to Go

Well, I officially survived my second round of chemo infusions. Now, I am just dealing with the side effects for a few days and then I should be feeling good again until the next treatment in two weeks. Today they disconnected the pump and gave me the injection to encourage blood cell production. I have been napping off and on all afternoon and evening.

I am thankful to be free from carrying the pump around, and thankful that I have only been slightly queasy. I am thankful for sweet friends who have been bringing meals to us, running errands for me, and bringing supplies from the grocery store. They are awesome and will never really know how much the small things mean to us, especially when we are unable or too tired to do them for ourselves.

The word of the day is "diarrhea." It has been in full swing since Tuesday night. We are praying that I will be able to control this with medication. I can dehydrate quickly with the ileostomy. I am also sore to the touch around my ribs, my neck, shoulders, back, chest, and arms. The ache seems to be spreading. The doctor told me to expect to have this for about forty-eight hours.

Hopefully I will feel better by the weekend.

Friday October 23, 2009
Pity Party

Thursday. Mark is at the gym. I am resting. Diarrhea and nausea are under control. I am trying to eat, but nothing sounds good or tastes right. My body still aches, even with Motrin, but the pain seems to be decreasing. I feel very weak and tired. I can fall asleep any time I close my eyes.

Without thinking, I put a piece of ice in my mouth. It feels like fire, and I spit it out across the kitchen! So many side effects, so many things to remember when I can barely remember my name anymore.

The tears come. I don't feel like I can do this. I'm not strong enough. What if it comes back? I'll never survive that. Dear Jesus, it's just You and me. And I can't do it, so it's really just You. I need You today.

I know in my mind that it is expected that I will still feel badly for a couple of days after the pump is disconnected as my body is processing and getting rid of the chemicals, but somehow I keep hoping that each new day I will suddenly not feel sick. I guess I set myself up for this.

Friday morning. I slept great. I am lying in bed. I feel good. I don't want to move. I don't want this good feeling to be replaced by something else. Maybe if I just stay in bed all day, just skip

Friday, and get up on Saturday.

The tears come again. A full-blown pity party! Lord, please help me to get my eyes on You. I know You are here.

Geoff Moore's song "He Knows My Name" comes on the radio:

"I have a Maker
He formed my heart
Before even time began
My life was in His hands

I have a Father
He calls me His own
He'll never leave me
No matter where I go

He knows my name
He knows my every thought
He sees each tear that falls
And hears me when I call"

I know You are here! Thank You for never leaving. Thank You for carrying me today.

"These trials will show that your faith is genuine. It is being tested as fire tests and purifies gold – though your faith is far more precious than mere gold. So when your faith remains strong through many trials, it will bring you much praise and glory and honor on the day when Jesus Christ is revealed to the whole world." 1 Peter 1:7 (NLT)

"You are building up an unshakable faith. Be furnishing the quiet places of your soul now. Fill them with all that is harmonious and good, beautiful, and enduring. Home-build in the Spirit now, and the waiting time will be well spent." – (God Calling)

Saturday October 24, 2009
What a Difference a Day Makes!

I have felt much better today, physically and emotionally. I am still tired but improving. Today I have also experienced tingling of my mouth, lips, and left arm and hand. This is a common and expected side effect of one of my chemo drugs.

I have continued to rest today and to stay out of circulation of the general human population. We are being extra careful to prevent exposure to swine flu or any of the other viruses that are going around the area. I will have my blood levels checked on Wednesday to see if the bone marrow-boosting injection has done what it's supposed to do. Then maybe I'll venture out to the grocery store. Exciting life, huh?

I did give myself a gold star today for ileostomy care and maintenance. I was not too excited when the doctor first told me that I would need a temporary ileostomy; but I want you to know that it has not been nearly as dreadful as I first imagined. Taking care of it has become routine. It's funny how we adjust to new things and then before long they seem to be a normal part of our lives. One of my initial concerns was the possibility of the skin around the stoma breaking down due to leaking digestive enzymes. I am very proud to tell you that my stoma is perfectly healthy, and the skin on my abdomen is intact without a hint of injury. I consider this to be an answer to my fearful prayers and I am thankful that God has taken good care of this.

One of the things I am most thankful for is all of my faithful friends. Their constant prayers and words of encouragement mean the world to me. They give me strength to keep walking this path and I will never be able to repay them. I am trusting that God will bless each one for their kindness and faithfulness toward me, and for seeing me through a difficult week.

Tuesday October 27, 2009
Hair Today, Gone Tomorrow

Before I started IV chemotherapy the oncologist told me that he didn't expect me to lose my hair. Good, I thought, because I didn't really want to lose my hair. I think if I had no hair I would look like a mouse or a bird. Then the oncologist said, "Your hair may thin some."

That was the understatement of the year! My hair is coming out all over the place! I am constantly plucking long blonde hairs off of my arms and shoulders. They are all over the couch, of course, and they cover the seat in Mark's car. Every time I wash my hair, or brush my hair, or run my hands through my hair, I come away with handfuls of hair. The last time I spoke at the church I happened to glance down at the stage and saw long blond hairs on the black carpet surrounding my stool. (I'd like to clarify that "stool" in this instance refers to a piece of furniture that you sit on. I know with my diagnosis and the frequent topics of my life that it could have been misinterpreted as another form of "stool.") My hair is everywhere! I guess I have more than I thought I had because I still have a good bit on my head, but if it keeps up like this, I may not have it for long.

I have always had long blond hair. It is a part of me. I'm not sure what I'd do without it. I'm not sure how I feel about wearing a wig, but it could actually be fun to shop for hats! And since it will be the fall and winter season, hats would be useful. I doubt it will come to that, but I do know that over the next few months my hair will continue to grow thinner, my roots will continue to grow out, and my gray hairs will start to show themselves. Please be kind to me when you see this happening! It's not that I haven't gone to get my hair touched up; it's just that I can't. Not until I am finished with chemo treatments. In the meantime I will try to keep my chin up, smile, and endure with dull, dry, brittle, thin, two-tone graying hair!

Thursday October 29, 2009
Blood Count Update

I saw the oncologist today and had my blood drawn, again. My blood counts are still low, which was expected as a result of my last chemo treatment. However they have not dropped as low as they did after the first treatment. My total white blood cell count was 2.8 today. It needs to be 3.0 in order for me to safely receive my next chemo treatment on Monday. The neutrophil count was 0.82 today and it needs to get up to 1.0. The doctor is confident that the levels will be where we need them to be by Monday. Please keep praying that they will. In the meantime, I will continue to quarantine myself as much as possible. It's no fun to be home all the time missing my friends, and missing out on so many things. But, on the positive side, my desk is now clean, stacks of paperwork are getting filed, and the kitchen counters have been cleared off. My closet can't be far behind... or... maybe it can!

Friday October 30, 2009
Thankfulness

Lately, I've had a lot of time to myself, time alone and time to think. Thinking can be good, but sometimes it can lead down roads of discouragement and despair. Occasionally, in order to keep my thinking in the real world, I like to take the time to write down things for which I am thankful. I don't just make a quick, short list of the top ten things. That's too easy, and would probably always include the same top ten. Instead I challenge myself to make a list of one hundred things for which I am thankful. It starts with the usual things – my husband, my family, my friends, my church – but by the time I get to one hundred, I am listing things that I rarely think of:

- Thank You God for creating eyelashes to protect my eyes.
- Thank You God for allowing me to win the spelling bee in 4th grade.
- Thank You God for the hummingbirds that come to our yard every year.
- Thank You God for indoor plumbing.
- Thank You God that the roach crawled on Mark in the night and not on me.

So many things to be thankful for, and yet I rarely take the time to express my gratitude.

Psychologist Dr. Brenda Shoshanna said the following:

"There is one sure fire medicine which cures all pain and opens the way for your greater good. It allows you to sleep well at night, wake up refreshed and filled with enthusiasm for your daily tasks. This medicine is abundantly available, has no side effects and can be taken in large or small doses regularly. You need no one to prescribe it. The more you take, the sweeter it is. The medicine is the practice of thankfulness." (Shoshanna, Dr. Brenda. "The Power of Thankfulness." 55-*Alive*, Target Directories Corp! October 30, 2009.)

Thankfulness changes us. It changes our thinking. It changes our attitude. It changes our outlook on life. The more we practice thankfulness, the deeper it seeps into our being and transforms us.

I've heard thankfulness defined as "the expression of joy Godward," which explains the power of thankfulness perfectly. When we express our gratitude toward God, He uses it to transform our lives.

I challenge you today to sit down and write out 100 things for which you are thankful. It will change you.

"And let the peace that comes from Christ rule in your hearts... And always be thankful." Colossians 3:15 (NLT)

"Do you see what we've got? An unshakable kingdom! And do you know how thankful we must be? Not only thankful, but brimming with worship, deeply reverent before God." Hebrews 12:28 (The Message)

Sunday November 1, 2009
Tragedy Strikes

Tragedy strikes. No one is exempt. It comes swiftly, surprising those who are touched, leaving bewilderment and shock in its wake. As I get older I am realizing that tragedy is a normal part of the human experience. In the last month alone I have been aware of the following:

- A four-year-old boy is diagnosed with a brain tumor.
- A 38 year old mother dies leaving a husband and three children.
- A 48 year old man is suddenly jobless after years of faithful work on the job.
- A father falls, breaking his neck, he struggles for life for six weeks, and then passes away.
- A son commits suicide, leaving his parents devastated and questioning.
- A young mother's breast cancer returns with a vengeance.

- A young preacher is killed in a head-on collision leaving his family fatherless and his church without a pastor.

How do we survive these kinds of things? Where do we go with our grief? Where do we take our questions, our anger, our pain, and our fear? I've stood by watching these stories be lived out and I've wondered how does someone survive that tragedy? And I've prayed. "God, be real to them. Be real to them. Let them feel Your presence."

My cancer diagnosis can't even compare to some of these other losses, but the one thing it has shown me is that God is real. He is here. He will never leave.

In our anguish we usually question "Why?" But I have found that this question never brings any comfort. And, honestly, if I knew why, would it really make me feel any better or lessen my grief or fill my emptiness? I don't think so.

Instead of looking for "why" I start looking for "who." Who is the one who said He would catch my tears in His hand and dry every tear from my eye, the one who said He would never leave me or forsake me, the one who said He would turn my mourning into dancing? He's the one who will see me through when tragedy strikes. He is the only one who can.

"The Lord is there to rescue all who are discouraged and have given up hope." Psalm 34:18 (CEV)

"He heals the brokenhearted and bandages their wounds." Psalm 147:3 (NLT)

Monday November 2, 2009
Chemo Round Three

My total white blood count today was 3.8 and my neutrophils were at 7.0. So, today began round three of chemotherapy. I am physically wiped out. Round three immediately began with nausea, fatigue, diarrhea, peripheral neuropathy, and muscle cramps in my hands and legs. The cramps are due to the chemo's effect on my electrolytes. It is not painful, but it is weird. I have a hard time controlling my fingers. It is followed the next few days by sleeping and recovering. Round three finishes with the usual expected side effects – ever-present nausea and diarrhea, hand and leg cramping, cold-sensitive mouth and throat, tingling lips, twitching eyes, hiccups, fatigue, and aching bones. The good news is that I know it is only a matter of a few days and then I will be feeling much better. And the even better news is that I am now officially one quarter of the way finished with my chemotherapy treatments! I am so grateful for the faithful prayers that have been whispered on my behalf.

Thursday November 5, 2009
I Hate Cancer

I hate cancer and I hate chemotherapy. That pretty much sums up my week. Today was day four of feeling sick and having an assortment of weird, disconcerting side effects. Not only do the chemicals affect every cell of my body, they seem to creep into my mind and emotions as well. I can see that the next five months are going to be a tough mental and emotional battle for me as well as being a physical one.

Mark and I had a good friend, Rich, when we lived in Fort Worth. Whenever Rich was sick he would say he felt like "death eating a cracker." I used to laugh at that statement, but now I completely understand what "death eating a cracker" feels like! Another friend told me that she called chemotherapy "chemo-sobby" because she cried all the time. I am definitely living in chemo-sobby land! The sad thing is that I feel so sick I want to cry, but it hurts too much to cry. Even the bones in my face hurt.

One of the most relaxing things for me is to sit outside in the sun. I haven't been able to do this since I began this whole journey due to the drugs I am taking. My skin is more sensitive to the sun and can burn and damage easily. The last few days we have had perfect weather in Houston. This is not the norm and I was so sad to be sitting inside, again, and missing out on such beautiful days. So today I decided to go outside and enjoy the weather, thinking it might help me to feel better.

I positioned myself in one of our lounge chairs, covered myself from head to toe with clothing and towels, completely protecting myself from the sun. There's no telling what my neighbors thought, but it sure felt good to hear the trickle of the water from the fountains, to hear the birds singing, to feel the warmth of the sun, and to feel the gentle breeze! The breeze even blew up under the towel over my head and I knew it was God reminding me of His presence with me.

The simple things in life are sweet. I am looking forward to a better tomorrow.

Saturday November 7, 2009
Fun Times!

Mark and I attended an awards luncheon on Friday. I was honored to be recognized alongside four other leaders in our community. I was especially thankful to have my parents and my brother Cary with me, as well as some of my sweet friends. They gave me the strength I needed to be there while still recovering from chemotherapy.

My special prayer for the day was that I would not vomit when I went up to receive the award. Thankfully, my queasy stomach remained calm. The only issue I had besides fatigue was the drawing up of the muscles in my hands and legs. I had trouble actually cutting my food and feeding myself, which was kind of comical. Then, as I stood at the side of the platform waiting to be called up to receive the award, I was just hoping that my legs would actually cooperate and I would be able to climb the steps and hold the award with my hands and not grab it with my arms! Thankfully, everything turned out fine and we all had a nice time. One of the sweetest parts of the whole day was that my mother had the privilege of saying the opening prayer. When she did she shared the following verse: *"Because he bends down to listen, I will pray as long as I have breath!" Psalm 116:2 (NLT)*

Isn't that a beautiful picture of God's love for us? He bends down to listen! What an amazing promise we can hold on to. And what a great gift to know that my mom is praying for me!

Sunday November 8, 2009
Precious Thoughts

A sweet friend of mine sent me a note the other day and she ended it with these words, "God hears your name constantly before Him."

That simple sentence brought such strength and encouragement to me. I am awestruck that the God of the universe would think about me at all, and yet I know that He does. I am reminded of this truth all the time.

"How precious are your thoughts about me, O God. They cannot be numbered!" Psalm 139:17 (NLT)

Did you hear that? They cannot be numbered! He thinks about me so much that it's impossible to count His thoughts. Nothing escapes His notice – not my fatigue or frustration, not my freaky side effects, not the days ahead that He has already planned. Nothing. He is thinking about me day and night. He knows what my white blood cell count is doing, He knows how many days I will feel sick to my stomach, He knows about each muscle twitch before it happens!

And He is thinking of the good days ahead too – the day I finish my last chemo treatment, the day I change my last ileostomy bag, the day I get to eat ice cream again, the day I celebrate His goodness and faithfulness with my friends in Costa Rica, and the day I finally visit the village of Matara in Burundi, Africa. God is thinking of these things because He is thinking of me. My God is good.

I hope you will start your week meditating on the fact that His thoughts about you cannot be numbered.

Monday November 9, 2009
View from the Exam Table

I had a check-up with the surgeon today. As I reclined on the exam table I took note of the various things in the room: calming artwork, the doctor's headgear and headlamp for peering into unseen worlds, rubber tubes and medical instruments of torture, the doctor's gloves (Why he needs "diamond grip" gloves, I don't want to know.), and my faithful husband, waiting with me yet again. A fun time was had by all! Can you hear the sarcasm? Thankfully, everything is healing as expected.

Mark and I walked out of the office building and suddenly I was sobbing. I felt like my body could just dissolve in a heap! I realized that I had kept myself steeled for the past week through chemotherapy, side effects, Friday's luncheon, helping Mark prepare for the weekend, and my appointment today. Finally, the tension let go and I was a mess. We stopped to pick up lunch and when we got home Mark collapsed on the couch and slept soundly for a couple of hours. I think he was feeling the same things I felt. Cancer is exhausting for everyone.

Tuesday November 10, 2009
Amazing Day

I had the most amazing day today!

I am learning to appreciate the small things every day, like waking up and not feeling sick. That is an incredible feeling that I most often take for granted. I hope I will remember to be thankful for each day of good health long after this battle is over.

I spent the morning with a friend and her six-week-old daughter. What a fun time of snuggling and playing with a very special little baby! Thank you, God, for new life, and for letting me be a part of this one.

Later I walked down to get the mail and there was a package from my dad's cousin, Mary. I was so excited when I saw it; it felt like Christmas. The package said, "Do not bend," and I knew! Mary is an artist. She paints beautiful pictures of flowers, landscapes, and outdoor scenes. I knew this package contained something special. When I opened the package I found a beautiful print of her painting "Afternoon Glories" and a copy of the Serenity Prayer, and a very sweet note from Mary. My grandmother kept a small plaque of the Serenity Prayer in her bathroom. It was there my whole life. It was how she chose to live her life every day. Mary knew this, and she sent me this prayer as an encouragement in my battle with cancer. The tears came again; tears for my grandmother, tears for the sweet love

of a cousin, and tears of gratitude for God who is carrying me
through.

"God grant me the serenity to accept the things I cannot change,
the courage to change the things I can, and the wisdom to know
the difference." (Anonymous)

Wednesday November 11, 2009
Laura's Song

So far, every step of this journey has been bathed in music. From
those pre-diagnosis days when I awoke every night with lyrics
playing in my head, to the crisis moments when God would meet
me with a particular song on the radio. This is nothing new for
me. I have always related to God through music.

For the past few months the worship team at our church has
been working on producing the third Community of Faith worship
album. Donald and one of the worship team members, Amos
Rivera, were inspired to write a song from some of the Scriptures
and writings I had shared with them from my cancer journey thus
far. The first time I heard the song I just cried. It is beautiful and
it expresses so well the emotions I've felt and the desire of my
heart.

"When my world comes crashing down and I am facing death,
I will rest again for You are good to me.
Lord, I trust You are my strength in times that I am weak.
So, I thank You for the chance to live what I believe
Simply knowing how You love is bringing such a peace
But there is more to this than knowing what could be
I have access to Your pow'r, you've given me the keys
Now I have the faith to stand and live what I believe
You give me life, you're saving me

All through the night I will sing Your songs of praise
I know You will never leave me
Thank You for the chance to live what I believe
Let my life be the proof of the hope found in You."
("Live What I Believe," by Donald Butler and Amos Rivera)
God, thank You again, for the music of life.

Thursday November 12, 2009

I went to the doctor yesterday and the news was good. I had a
normal white blood cell count. My platelets are low, but they
should be back up by Monday in time for me to receive my fourth
chemo treatment. That's all good, but can I tell you how sick I
am of going to doctors' offices? I make up to three visits to doctor
offices every week. And I don't want to go anymore.

I so wish I could go back to my old life, but I know that
that will never happen. Everything has changed. Things will
eventually settle down and they will probably be better, but
they will never be the same. I am different. Mark is different.
Our relationship is different. Our thinking is different. All for the
better I'm sure, but it's painful to change. There is grief in the
process, even when the changes are good ones. I just want to be
on the other side of this.

As I was thinking all these thoughts today I came across a
verse of Scripture that I've probably read a thousand times, but
for some reason today it really spoke to me.

"For in him we live and move and have our being." Acts 17:28 (NIV)

I am never outside of His presence. Ever. I live in His presence.
I move in His presence. My very being comes to life in His
presence. How cool is that? Every time I go to the doctor I am
surrounded by His presence. Every time I run to the bathroom
I am surrounded by His presence. Every time I swallow a pill I
am surrounded by His presence. Every time they infuse crazy

chemicals into my body I am surrounded by His presence. Every tear I cry, He feels. Every hope or wish or dream I have, He knows. Every loss, every painful readjustment of my life, every thing I've missed out on in the last six months, He has been there. Filtering everything that comes into my life through His fingers of love. I am never outside of His presence. I will make it through this, because in His presence I live and move and have my being.

Saturday November 14, 2009
Life-transforming Friendship

Two years ago at our church we began a partnership with the Batwa people of Burundi, Africa. This partnership has turned into a life-transforming friendship for the Batwa as well as for the people of Community of Faith. We have learned so much from them about community, about gratitude, about sharing, about perseverance, about worship, and about hope. Sometimes God's blessings and teachings come in the most unexpected ways and in the most unexpected places! We know God is going to do great things as we continue to grow deeper in friendship with our Batwa family.

My road probably won't lead me to Burundi this year, but in spite of that, God has definitely been teaching me about friendship, love, perseverance, and hope right here at home. Just today a sweet friend brought me homemade gingerbread cookies to help calm my stomach during chemotherapy this week. It is amazing what the thoughtfulness and kindness of a friend can do to strengthen your spirit! These cookies will definitely be going with me tomorrow as I head back to the doctor's office in the morning.

I begin my fourth round of chemotherapy Monday morning, and honestly, I am dreading it. I don't look forward to feeling sick and exhausted all week. I don't look forward to drawing blood and needle sticks. For several days I have been fighting a mental battle in preparation for this week. When I even think about walking into the infusion room I immediately feel nauseous. I am trusting that all my friends are praying for me this week. Praying for physical, emotional, mental, and spiritual strength. Praying that I will recognize God's presence with me and that I will trust in His goodness. Praying that God will shine through me every day. Praying that I will learn this lesson of perseverance and faith.

The doctor is planning to give me a new anti-nausea medication this round. I have heard from other cancer survivors that this medication should knock out the nausea, so I am praying that it works as well for me as it has for others.

Thank you, to all of you, for teaching me what it means to truly be a friend, and what it means to be the Body of Christ.

"There is no room in love for fear..." 1 John 4:18 (*The Message*) Lord, please help me not to fear.

Sunday November 15, 2009
Polish Your Weapons

Tonight as I was sitting around dreading Monday I was reminded that I am in a war and I have an enemy.

"The thief's purpose is to steal and kill and destroy..." John 10:10 (*NLT*)

So, I thought I better polish my weapons for the fight. I spent the next hour putting together all the Scripture verses that God has led me to over these past six months. I am taking them with me to chemotherapy this week so that I can meditate on them while I'm there. I've even decided to try to memorize one verse each week. This is my verse for this week: *"But as for me, I trust in You."* Psalm 55:23 (*NIV*)

It's pretty simple, but I think if I carry this verse in my mind this week it could make significant changes in the way the week goes.

"For though we live in the world, we do not wage war as the world does. The weapons we fight with are not the weapons of the world."
2 Corinthians 10:3-4 (NIV)

Tuesday November 17, 2009
Chemo Round Four

The song "Live What I Believe" played in my head all night Sunday and was playing in my head all Monday morning before I left to go get chemo. I like how God does that for me.

Monday was a rough day. Thankfully, the new anti-nausea medication seems to be working. However, it is known that the effects of chemo are cumulative, normally getting more severe with each treatment. For me, that meant that by the time I left the doctor's office my muscles were already drawing up. My hands do weird contortions that are out of my control. My calf muscles are tight. When we finally got home, I wasn't sure I would be able to get out of the car. I made it out but had a lot of difficulty walking. I couldn't bend my legs or lift my feet off the ground. My feet were turning in. So, I shuffled along, like the Bride of Frankenstein, and made it to the couch where I immediately fell fast asleep. Later I washed my hands and discovered a new side effect. The temperature of the tap water let me know that the nerves in my hands are now feeling the effects of the chemo. It felt like electric shocks all over my hands. Touching anything cold causes this reaction - a doorknob, a handle, a glass, the computer keyboard. I now type with very nice purple gloves on my hands! The next few months should be interesting.

The good news is I am one day closer to done; and the weapons of my warfare have divine power! I am so thankful for the unseen battle being waged in prayer for me.

Today a friend share with me a poem written on the wall of a Nazi concentration camp after the captives were liberated. I am hanging onto these words for the times when I am waiting on the Lord.

I believe in the sun, even when it is not shining.
I believe in love, even when I do not feel it.
I believe in God, even when He is silent.

Thursday November 19, 2009

The last seventy-two hours were spent either sleeping in a chemo infusion chair, sleeping on the couch, or sleeping in my bed. Upon waking Thursday morning I close my eyes and wish I could sleep the next seventy-two hours and wake up next week instead. Before getting out of bed I run a few tests. Am I able to open my eyes? I couldn't open them Monday afternoon due to issues with muscle control. The eyes are working. Next I check the hands and feet for numbness and tingling. Do they move when I command them to? Can I bend my legs? Everything seems to be working this morning. I check the ileostomy for diarrhea. Yes, it's back, as expected.

I get out of bed. I am wearing sweat pants, sweat shirt, gloves, and socks. This is my protection from the nighttime cold to prevent my nerves from sending needles into my hands, feet, and legs.

I swallow pills with water heated in the microwave. My stomach seems to be calm so I drink a little more hot water (you can just imagine how refreshing this is) knowing that I am dehydrated and need to get as much fluid in my body as possible. There is nothing worse than drinking heated Gatorade or Pedialyte.

My stomach remains calm, so I decide to try breakfast. I get it down and return to my spot on the couch. The pets jump up to join me. They like all the warm clothes and blankets! All four of us drift off on the couch with the television quietly playing in the background.

When I wake up again, the dreaded nausea has returned. It seems to be a kind of motion sickness. If I don't move I feel relatively OK, but the moment I stand up I am nauseous. I gag often, but nothing comes up. Thankfully, the pharmacist has made an anti-nausea compound that can be rubbed on my wrists, bypassing the stomach and knocking out the nausea. It knocks me out too, and I sleep more.

With each treatment the side effects seem to hang around longer. This doesn't really give me encouragement for the next eight treatments. I don't like this. I wonder if I can really do eight more. I am clinging to my verse of the week:

"But as for me, I trust in you." Psalm 55:23 (NIV)

I start to cry again, but it is physically painful to do so. I have so many tears inside that can't find a way out.

Cancer is an awful disease. Every week I see so many people suffering as they fight for their lives. Many are elderly, some are young, some have been fighting for years and years. For some it has become a chronic disease, they continue to receive chemo treatments for months and years, just to keep the tumors at bay. I honestly cannot imagine how they do it.

I pray daily that no one else in my family or extended family ever has to fight this battle.

"The Lord will fight for you; you need only to be still." Exodus 14:14 (NIV)

Saturday November 21, 2009
Still Standing

Chemo round four – I win!

It is Saturday morning. I have been through a huge physical, emotional, mental, and spiritual battle this week. But I woke up this morning with the knowledge that I am still standing. I am weak and exhausted, but I survived round four!

So many friends have been the hands, feet, and voice of Jesus to me this week. I honestly believe that I would not have survived without them. They came alongside me just when I needed them. They gave me rides, watched over me as I slept, held my hand, gave me hugs, brought me flowers, spoke encouraging words, enticed me to drink fluids, and brought me food at the exact moment that I needed it. I am convinced that if not for these friends I would not have eaten all week. I just didn't have the strength or motivation to do so. I believe they gave life to me this week. God used them and I have been blessed because of it.

And so many have spoken and prayed Scripture over me. They continue to stand in the gap for me. When I think of these prayer warriors I am overwhelmed by their love. There are no words to express what is in my heart and what they do for me on a daily basis.

I have listened to worship music over and over, letting God's truth wash over me. This morning, as I find myself still standing after round four, I am reminded of the lyrics of one of those songs, "The Stand" by Hillsong:

"So I'll stand with arms high and heart abandoned in awe of the One who gave it all.
So I'll stand, my soul Lord to You abandoned, all I am is yours."

I can't raise my arms very high for very long at this point, but my heart and soul are abandoned to You, Lord. Thank you for seeing me through this week. Thank You for your mercy and Your grace. Thank You that when I am weak, You are strong.

I am still standing.

Sunday November 22, 2009
Side Benefits

Little-known side benefits of chemotherapy:

- You can stay in your pajamas all day (or all week!) and no one thinks less of you.
- You don't have to brush your hair – no one cares.
- You can fall asleep at any time, making napping very easy.
- You have no short-term memory – this can be bad, but it can also be a good thing!
- The hair on your legs and under your arms stops growing – no need to shave.
- You always have a good excuse for anything.
- Lifetime Membership in the I Survived Cancer and Cancer Treatment Club.
- You develop a deep empathy for all those fighting cancer.
- You meet the most amazing, strong, courageous people along the way.

"I lift up my eyes to the hills—where does my help come from? My help comes from the LORD, the Maker of heaven and earth" Psalm 121:1-2 (NIV)

Monday November 23, 2009
Rehydrated and It Feels So Good!

I can honestly say that the last week was the worst I've ever felt in my life. Granted, that's not really saying much because I've rarely been sick in my life! I had pneumonia when I was ten, and I get migraine headaches, but other than that, I just haven't been sick. So, this has been a whole new thing for me.

Thursday, Friday, and Saturday I was so weak that I rarely moved from my spot on the couch, and I continued to sleep away the hours. Apparently most of this weakness has been due to my inability to take in enough fluid to remain hydrated. Today I spent four hours at the doctor's office where they drew blood for lab tests and infused two liters of IV fluids. That's a lot of fluid pumped into my thirsty system! My body was so low on fluids that I didn't even need to go to the bathroom after having that amount of liquid added to my circulation. I felt much better afterward, and everyone agreed I definitely looked better! I'm not sure that's saying much either at this point.

We are looking forward to Thanksgiving with all our kids, family, and a few special friends. I know that having everyone home has the potential to tire me out, but I think the strength of being surrounded by family will overshadow anything else. I am looking forward to lots of laughs and hugs and making new memories.

Thursday November 26, 2009
Thanksgiving

The holidays have arrived and I still have cancer. I was trying to think of something profound to say about Thanksgiving or gratefulness. But I don't have anything. All I know is that I am grateful to be alive. I am grateful for the sounds of laughter in my house. I am grateful for the scent of pies cooking in the kitchen. I am grateful for books scattered on the kitchen table. I am grateful for my husband and my children. I am grateful for my family. I am grateful for the love that has been showered on us this year. I am grateful for amazing, compassionate doctors and nurses. I am grateful for my faithful friends. I am grateful for my church. I am grateful for the chance to see the Body of Christ in action. I am grateful for all the things I am learning.

More than anything, I am grateful to be a daughter of the King of Kings and Lord of Lords. I am grateful that He knows me and He loves me completely. I am grateful that He never leaves me. I am grateful that when I am weak, He is strong. There is no other God above Him and I will serve Him and praise Him forever.

"So remember this and keep it firmly in mind: The Lord is God both in heaven and on earth, and there is no other." Deuteronomy 4:39 (NLT)

"Blessing and glory and wisdom and thanksgiving and honor and power and strength belong to our God forever and ever! Amen." Revelation 7:12 (NLT)

Sunday November 29, 2009
He Is for Me

I go back to the oncologist tomorrow to begin treatment number five. It would be an understatement to say that I am not looking forward to this week. In fact, I have been dreading it since the end of my last treatment. It is a constant battle in my mind to choose peace, to choose to trust, and to choose to submit my desires and my life to God's hands. It seems like it should be so easy. Knowing who God is and knowing how much He loves me, I still struggle.

The crazy thing is that even through my struggle I have found Him here, faithfully calling out to me and giving His strength and encouragement to me. For the past seventy-two hours the song "You Are For Me" by Kari Jobe has been playing non-stop in my head. Every time I wake up in the night the lyrics are still going through my head. At first I thought this is just a song that I like so I am singing it. And then I realized that it wasn't me. God was singing it to me. He has been reminding me that I can trust Him with this treatment and with this week. He is for me. He will be here. Whatever happens, however I feel, He will be here and carry me through.

"So faithful, So constant, So loving and so true
So powerful in all You do
You fill me, You see me, You know my every Move
You love for me to sing to You
I know that You are for me, I know that you are for me
I know that You will never forsake me in my weakness
I know that You have come down, Even if to write upon
    my heart
To remind me who You are
So patient, So gracious, So merciful and true
So wonderful in all You do
You fill me, You see me, You know my every move
You love for me to sing to You
I know that You are for me, I know that you are for me
I know that You will never forsake me in my weakness
I know that You have come down, even if to write upon my
    heart
To remind me who you are"
("You Are For Me," by Kari Jobe)

He is for me. That's all I need.

Monday November 30, 2009
Early Christmas Present

You never know what a day will bring. After all my dread leading up to today, I woke up with perfect peace. I know that is a result of the prayers of those who love me. We went to the oncologist today expecting to begin treatment number five. Unfortunately my platelet count was too low and I was unable to receive the treatment. I don't like having to postpone treatments, but I feel like I got a reprieve this week - one more week to feel good.

And then the oncologist gave me the best early Christmas present ever! He told us that we would be doing eight treatments and not twelve! Current research is showing that in cases like mine eight treatments are effective. That means I am now halfway done with chemotherapy! I am so happy I can hardly stand it! If I stay on schedule then I should finish by late January or early February.

They are also planning to give me lots of IV fluids with the next treatment, and to set up home health for me so that I can give myself IV fluids in between treatments. This will keep me from becoming dehydrated like last time, which will make Mark and I both feel better. As rough as the last treatment was for me, it was even harder for Mark to watch.

God is for me!

Saturday December 5, 2009
Love Is What Will Remain

This week has been such a gift to me. Obviously God knew that I needed an extra week to rest before my next chemo treatment. My tendency, when I am feeling good, is to overdo it. So, I have been forcing myself to rest this week even though I am feeling good. I figured that if God gave me an extra week to rest then I better rest. He knows what I need.

I have also taken this week to get everything ready for Christmas. I finished my Christmas shopping (most of it online), wrapped the gifts, worked on the annual Christmas letter, and sorted through several piles of papers that have been growing over the last several months.

For the most part, I have felt well. But there are moments when the fatigue still hits, and almost every evening I feel a twinge of nausea. I look forward to the day that I have a normal energy level and no more digestive tract issues. That day is coming, and it's even sooner than we thought!

God continues to encourage me through so many friends. I received an email today from my friend Paul. He has experienced a lot of difficult things in his life and his honest email brought me to tears. I love his words.

"The truth about the tumultuous nature of the world God brought us to is one of only two things I know to be certain. The other is that God is here always and is in control. ONLY He is in control. See, the greatest lesson He wants us to learn is how to accept His unconditional love and pass it on to every human we encounter. He wants it to be like reflex. But the only way to teach us to rely on His unconditional love in a way we will never forget, that we might share it with the world AND with ourselves, in every moment we have a breath in our lungs... is to shake us so hard and so loose, that everything falls out of our pockets, off of our bodies, leaving us clinging to two truths: 1. The world will always storm and shake. 2. Love is what will remain."

Sunday December 6, 2009
Unspeakable Joy! Sunday

The most amazing thing has happened to me. Although the last seven months have been some of the hardest months to live through for me, I have also experienced the most constant joy that I have ever experienced in my life. It seems like such a contradiction to have received a life-threatening diagnosis and yet to find constant joy in the midst of it all. I've shared before that I am not naturally a positive person; I tend to be melancholy and to see the negative side of things. But it's as if that has all disappeared in the last seven months and been replaced by a deep joy that bubbles up from inside of me every day. Not at all what I would have expected as a side effect of cancer!

I read this statement recently from Sarah Young in her book *Jesus Calling*:

"During times of severe testing, even the best theology can fail you if it isn't accompanied by experiential knowledge of Me. The ultimate protection against sinking during life's storms is devoting time to develop your friendship with Me."

I think this is the source of my joy. In the last seven months I have come to know my creator more deeply than ever before. And I have let Him know me. I have talked to Him, argued with Him, cried to Him, rested in His arms, waited for Him, trusted Him, and followed Him blindly. As our intimacy with each other has grown, my awareness and understanding of His deep love for me has washed over everything. It has covered everything, and colored everything. Knowing what I now know, I don't think it is possible to experience a day without joy.

One of my favorite things about the Christmas season is singing Christmas carols. I have them playing constantly in the house, and I love singing them at church. Today we sang an old standard, "Joy to the World." Chris Tomlin has added a new refrain to this carol and I was so happy to sing it out today!

"Joy, unspeakable joy
An overflowing well no tongue can tell
Joy, unspeakable joy
Rises in my soul, never lets me go."

That's the song of my heart, in the midst of cancer – unspeakable joy!

I hope you find this joy in your life.

"I have loved you with an everlasting love; I have drawn you with loving-kindness." Jeremiah 31:3 (NIV)

"Because of the Lord's great love we are not consumed, for His compassions never fail. They are new every morning; great is Your faithfulness. I say to myself, 'The Lord is my portion; therefore I will wait for Him.' The Lord is good to those whose hope is in Him, to the one who seeks Him; it is good to wait quietly for the salvation of the Lord." Lamentations 3:22-26 (NIV)

Tuesday December 8, 2009
From the Sidelines

When I was ten years old I had viral pneumonia. I was out of school for a whole month as we fought this disease. Two things from this experience have always stuck in my memory. One, the horrible taste of the medicated drops I had to put in the back of my throat – they smelled and tasted like vomit. I kind of think it was vomit, because it looked like it too. I'm not sure what the drug was, or what it was supposed to do, but I sure remember having to take it.

I also remember sitting in my bedroom and looking out my

window as the world seemed to pass me by. These were the days when all the kids in the neighborhood played together outside. Huge games of hide-n-seek, kick the can, and dodge ball. I remember being one of the dodge ball champions, not because I could throw the ball, because I certainly couldn't, but because I was small and quick and I could dodge the ball until the end. Every day I would watch while everyone was outside playing and I had to stay inside, resting, fighting viral agents trying to multiply in my system. It tore my heart out. I so longed to be outside with everyone else. I even wanted to go to school! Halloween came around and I missed going trick-or-treating. It was a ten-year-old's biggest disappointment.

Today I feel all those same things. I feel like I'm on the sidelines, wishing I could be in the game. I feel like I am missing out on so many things. Every year I look forward to the Ladies Christmas Dinner at our church. It is one of the most fun things we do all year. But tonight I won't be there. I'll be on the couch resting, fighting nausea, and wishing things could be different.

All those years ago as I listened to the doorbell ring repeatedly and children sing out "Trick-or-Treat!" I learned a most valuable lesson; a lesson in love and selflessness; a lesson in thoughtfulness; a lesson in compassion. As it was getting later on Halloween night the doorbell rang one last time. No one sang out "Trick-or-Treat." Instead it was a group of my dearest friends. As they went from door to door that night, they each carried an extra bag; Laura's bag. They told my story of pneumonia to all the neighbors and collected Halloween candy for me, and they were there to deliver it to me. That was the kindest act of friendship I had ever received. I have remembered their kindness all my life.

I know that even now as I sit on the sidelines, God is teaching me valuable lessons that I will carry through the rest of my life. May I be diligent in learning them; and may I be as compassionate as my ten year old friends!

"The Lord will make a way for you where no foot has been before. That which, like a sea, threatens to drown you, shall be a highway for your escape." Charles H. Spurgeon

Friday December 11, 2009

It's Friday! I survived to Friday! Round five was much better than round four. Still not fun, but much better. I did not have the issues with electrolyte imbalance and dehydration like I did last time, so I did not have the weird muscle contractions that always freak me out. That was a very pleasant relief.

I was given a shot of a long lasting anti-diarrheal medication on Monday afternoon. I knew it would be bad because it was obvious that none of the nurses wanted to give me the injection! It actually didn't hurt that much when the nurse gave it to me, but she showed me the needle afterward. It was a big one! I was fine until Wednesday morning. I woke up Wednesday and it felt like I had been kicked in the rump by a horse! I was so incredibly sore - still am - but thankfully the medication did what it was supposed to do. No diarrhea. I kept my electrolytes. No muscle weirdness. Emotional relief.

I also had a home health nurse come to the house this week to set me up to give myself IV fluids and electrolytes for three days. This was much needed and much appreciated as I ate and drank almost nothing Monday through Thursday. I now weigh two pounds more than I weighed when I got pregnant with our firstborn child. I don't recommend this diet plan. I am still extremely weak, but I am no longer retching up my intestines. I am resting and celebrating only three more treatments to go. My next treatment is scheduled for the week of Christmas.

"And I am convinced that nothing can ever separate us from God's

love. Neither death nor life, neither angels nor demons, neither our
fears for today nor our worries about tomorrow—not even the powers
of hell can separate us from God's love. No power in the sky above or
in the earth below—indeed, nothing in all creation will ever be able
to separate us from the love of God that is revealed in Christ Jesus our
Lord." Romans 8:38-39 (NLT)

Sunday December 13, 2009
Weekend at Laura's

I had a great weekend. I am still dealing with weakness and a few
other side effects, but in general I am feeling well.

One of the things I have missed most through this whole
ordeal is my weekends at church. We have four services at
Community of Faith and I normally attend all four. By the end of
the weekend I have Mark's sermon memorized. The weekends
after chemo treatments I am just too physically weak to go.
So, this being one of those weekends, I was feeling pretty sad
on Saturday afternoon. I knew that this weekend would be
special as we celebrated our annual "Give Your Best Gift to
Jesus" offering, baby dedication, and the Community of Faith
STOMP version of "The Little Drummer Boy," one of my favorite
Christmas traditions at the church! As Mark left the house
Saturday for the evening service I was in tears, wishing that I
could be a part of all that would happen this weekend.

As usually happens, God met me there. He whispered to my
heart that I did have a part in the weekend services; my part was
to pray. What a humbling thought that God would call on me to
pray for His church. The tears disappeared as I was immediately
energized and jumped right into my task. I spent the next hour
praying for God's power and His Spirit to fill Community of Faith,
and for each one in attendance to experience the love of Christ. I

prayed that every person at the church would be fully committed, body and soul - the same prayer I have been praying daily this year. What an amazing gift to be able to end the year praying for all the people I love so much who have been praying for me all these months.

I also had the freedom to belt out praise songs and Christmas carols at the top of my lungs with no one around to hear! I danced with the cat as we remembered God's precious gift to us at Christmas; and then I collapsed on the couch, energy spent, full of that "unspeakable joy." I may not have been physically present at church this weekend, but I was definitely there!

To top it all off, on Sunday, our amazing tech team set things up so that I could view one of the services live over the internet. I had a great view from the ledge of the sound booth in the back of the room! I didn't miss a thing. Isn't technology great? Thank You, God, for allowing me to still be a part, and thank you tech team for making it happen.

One of the lyrics that the worship team sang today says, "I will rest again for You are good to me." He has been good to me, even while I rest.

"For the Mighty One is holy, and He has done great things for me. He shows mercy from generation to generation to all who fear Him." Luke 1:49 (NLT)

Monday December 14, 2009
New Gutters

This story is based on a real life incident. Names have been changed to protect the innocent.

Scene:
New gutters are being put on the house. It takes a couple of days

to get the job done. The crew works all day Tuesday and then comes back Thursday morning to finish the job.

Characters:
Work Crew Leader: He is dressed in jeans, plaid flannel shirt, work boots and hat. He has a clipboard. He is in charge.

Suburban Housewife Fighting Cancer: She hasn't showered in four days. Her hair is in a four-day-old slept-in ponytail with a halo of hair sticking out all over her head, her skin is sallow. She wears no make-up, dark circles are evident under her eyes. She is wearing the same pajamas she's had on for four days, dirty socks, black gloves, and reading glasses.

Lighting:
The house is dark, lit only by the lights of the Christmas tree and the glow of the fire. Window blinds are closed.

Action:
9:00 a.m. Suburban Housewife Fighting Cancer is home alone, lying on the couch, again. Her goal for the day is not to move. Every move brings with it waves of nausea.

(Sound cue: doorbell rings)

Suburban Housewife: Not moving, she thinks to herself, "I will not answer the door. Whoever it is will go away."

(Sound cue: doorbell rings again)

Suburban housewife: Thinks to herself, "It must be someone who really needs something." She rises from the couch, gagging with each move of her body, wincing with the ache of her bones, and slowly shuffles to the front door. Forgetting her appearance, she opens the door...

Work Crew Leader: (seeing Suburban Housewife Fighting Cancer) Laughs out loud!

Suburban Housewife: (realizing how she looks) Laughs out loud too.

Work Crew Leader: (with big smile on his face, stuttering) "I am sorry..."

Suburban Housewife: (still laughing) "It's ok. I know."

Work Crew Leader: "We are here to finish the gutters."

Suburban Housewife: "That's great. Thank you."

Final Scene:
Gutters are in place. Work crew drives away, shaking their heads, wondering if there are other trolls who live in that house.

THE END

Wednesday December 16, 2009
Life Divided

It is interesting living a life that is divided into "every other week" intervals. Knowing that I will be sick and unable to accomplish anything during a chemo week, once my strength is improved I spend the off-week trying to get everything done that will need to be done in the next two weeks. This requires thought and planning... and memory. Sadly, my thinking, planning, and memory have been sorely impaired by the chemo treatments. I find myself making multiple lists (which is not really unusual for me), but then I constantly misplace the lists. I'm sure one day I will find them around the house and the car and get a good laugh.

This "every other week" life also produces a kind of frantic pace that I am sure is not how God intends for me to live. I catch myself talking to myself and telling me, "It's OK. You don't have to get everything done. You CAN'T get everything done. Relax. Rest. Relax. Rest. It's OK." So, if you see me out in the neighborhood looking lost, it's because I've misplaced my list, which is my brain; and if you see me frantically running around, please stop me and tell me to go home and REST!

"Be still in the presence of the Lord, and wait patiently for him to act." Psalm 37:7 (NLT)

"Let my soul be at rest again, for the Lord has been good to me." Psalm 116:7 (NLT)

I had an appointment with the surgeon today (Yes, it was just as fun as ever!). Everything is still healing well. He told me that if we actually finish chemo treatments the end of January then we can plan on surgery mid-February to close the ileostomy. I am beginning to see light at the end of the tunnel.

I am feeling well this week. I still tire easily and I have a few pesky side effects, in particular the nerve irritation in my hands and feet. They still can't tolerate anything cold. I wear gloves and socks 24/7. But, in the whole scheme of things that is a small inconvenience.

Top 10 Things it is Difficult to Do with Gloves on Your Hands:

1. Brush and floss your teeth
2. Wash your face
3. Put on make-up
4. Type on a computer

5. Crack eggs
6. Address and sign Christmas cards
7. Wrap Christmas gifts
8. Open canned cat food
9. Empty and/or change an ileostomy bag
10. Look fashionable

Thursday December 17, 2009
How Are You Feeling?

The first question I am asked by anyone who sees me is, "How are you feeling?" They ask out of genuine concern and affection, but I dread that question. I have discovered that I feel different each day, ranging from horribly sick to pretty well in a matter of a few days. It is a weird experience to feel like you are dying on a Thursday and then feel relatively normal by the following Tuesday; and then to have this cycle repeated every two weeks.

I have learned to answer the question for today.

Today I feel tired.

Today I feel better.

Today I feel awful.

Today I feel weak.

Today I feel angry.

Today I feel good.

Today. I am learning that this is exactly how God wants me to live my life. Live it today. I don't know how many years or months I have to live, and neither does anyone else. But I know I have today. What will I do today? Waste it being angry or resentful? Waste it feeling regret? Waste it in a fit of worry? Or will I make the most of the day God has given me? Every day brings opportunities to love someone, to forgive someone, to encourage someone, to provide for someone, to help someone. Am I looking for those opportunities and taking advantage of them? Lord, please keep reminding me to live today. Help me to see the opportunities You give me.

"This is the day the Lord has made..." Psalm 118:24 (NLT)

Monday December 21, 2009
Living Proof

I actually put my shoes on the wrong feet the other day. I haven't done that since I was three years old. They say that chemotherapy affects your brain. You can't remember things well; you can't recall names and words. They call this "chemo brain." It lasts throughout chemotherapy treatment and for some time afterward. Obviously, it has affected my brain. I told Mark that I have reverted to being a three year old. I put my shoes on the wrong feet and I use the bathroom in my pants! OK, it's in a bag, so it's not exactly the same, but still...

I was not able to receive my chemo treatment this week because my platelet count was too low. Normal platelet counts are 150,000 - 450,000. My platelet count today was 45,000. It needs to be at least 100,000 for me to safely receive chemotherapy. While I am disappointed that I won't be able to get one more treatment out of the way, I am happy that I won't be feeling sick on Christmas and that I will get to attend the Christmas Eve services at our church! There is nothing special I can do to increase my platelet count but continue to rest and eat well. With time, my bone marrow will eventually replace the platelets that have been lost. I return to the doctor next Monday to check my blood counts. If the platelets are back up then I will start my next treatment that day. Praying for a platelet count of at least 100,000 by Monday.

Friday December 25, 2009
How Divine His Goodness!

I've been reading through a book called *Meditations of a Hermit* by Charles de Foucauld. His words struck me as true this Christmas Day.

> *"God is good that he has so despoiled us of everything, that we can draw breath only by turning our heads towards him. How great is his mercy, how divine his goodness, for he has torn everything from us in order that we may be more completely his."*

Thank You, God, that You are pouring abundant grace into my soul.

Saturday December 26, 2009
The "Wonder" of Christmas

I had a great Christmas. It was nice not to be sick this week and to be able to enjoy time with family, friends, and with our church. But somehow all the recent "big events" - Thanksgiving, Graduation, Christmas – bring with them thoughts of wonder. Not the "wonder" of Christmas, but the "wonder" of cancer...

> I wonder how many more Thanksgivings I will share with my family?
> I wonder if I will see Ashley's graduation?
> I wonder if this will be my last Christmas?
> I wonder...

As I lay in bed on Christmas Eve, trying to fall asleep following five great services at Community of Faith, I was "wondering." And then music started playing in my head, an old hymn that I learned growing up. God's peace washed over me again as He reminded me that all is well. I can trust Him. No need to wonder anymore.

"Jesus, Jesus, how I trust Him, How I've proved Him o'er and o'er. Jesus, Jesus, Precious Jesus! O for grace to trust Him more." ("Tis So Sweet To Trust In Jesus," by Louisa M.R. Stead, 1882)

Lord, please give me the grace to trust You more. You have it all planned out and You only do what is best for me and for my family. You can't do anything else.

"...he remains faithful, for he cannot deny who he is." 2 Timothy 2:13 (NLT)

"In you our fathers put their trust; they trusted and you delivered them. They cried to you and were saved; in you they trusted and were not disappointed." Psalm 22:4-5 (NASB)

"Hold us in quiet through the age-long minute
While Thou art silent, and the wind is shrill:
Can the boat sink while Thou, dear Lord, art in it?
Can the heart faint that waiteth on Thy will?"
"Toward Jerusalem", Amy Carmichael

Sunday December 27, 2009
Remember

I woke up Christmas morning with a new song in my head, a traditional English Christmas Carol written by an unknown composer in the 1700s:

"God rest you merry, gentlemen,
Let nothing you dismay,
For Jesus Christ our Saviour
Was born upon this day."

Just those lines, repeating over and over in my brain. Funny how God uses music to communicate His truths to me, to comfort and encourage me, to prod me to trust Him, to believe Him.

As I lay there singing those two lines, it hit me again. My *Savior* was born on Christmas Day. I *have* a Savior! I don't have to wonder. I don't have to be dismayed. He *is* God. He IS in control. He has GOOD plans for me.

Thank You, God, for reminding me! Christ our Savior was born on Christmas Day! "*O tidings of comfort and joy, comfort and joy, O tidings of comfort and joy!*"

Monday December 28, 2009
Chemo Round Six

Thanks again to so many prayers, my blood levels were good today so we started round six! I am home now and resting until I go back tomorrow morning for day two of infusions. Again, everyone asks how I am feeling. I feel like I've had toxic chemicals pumped into my body! I feel like I am sick all over, and I am very tired; but thankfully I am not having any of the weird side effects related to electrolyte imbalance.

Tuesday December 29, 2009
Letter to My Kids, Just So You Know

Dear Ashley, Sarah, David, and Sydneyann,

Sorry for the recent melancholy posts, but you know how I am. It's in the genes! I just wanted to let you know that I plan to live to be 84! (Why 84? I don't know!) We will share so many Thanksgiving turkeys (and Tofurky!) together, and years of Christmas cookie making. I plan to be at Ashley's graduation shouting just as loudly as I did at David and Sarah's graduation (and would have at Sydneyann's if it hadn't been canceled by the ice storm!). I will be there when you walk down the aisle and marry the man of your dreams, and I will be holding your hand (if you want me to) as you labor and give birth to my grandchildren.

We will continue to travel the world, making memories, learning new things, and sharing the love of Christ along the way. I will text you random thoughts, and send you Halloween treat boxes. We will dream dreams, share secrets, dry each other's tears, and make crazy videos. I will be your biggest cheerleader, celebrating your every success! I will pray for you every day. I am so thankful for the gift of being your mother. I am cancer-free and plan to stay that way! Just so you know.

> Love,
> mom
> XOXOXOXO
> i.k.

Thursday December 31, 2009
Captive to Christ

I've spent most of the past four days sleeping. This round has seemed to go better than the others. Some say it's because I'm an old pro, and I guess there is some truth to that. I have learned over these weeks to just sleep, and keep sleeping, and let my body recover. I don't need to get up and try to get things done around the house. It can wait for next week.

But I have become convinced that although I may be an old pro, the difference this week has been due to something else.

With every treatment I have experienced extreme nausea. It is like a motion sickness. If I don't move, I don't feel it; but the moment I move my body I begin to gag and feel very sick. With every treatment I receive two IV drugs that combat nausea. They work on my digestive system. I also take a pill to combat nausea, which turns off the nausea receptors in my brain. I also have anti-nausea pills I can take at home as well as an anti-nausea compound that can be rubbed on my wrists. We shut off the nausea physically and mentally, but somehow I would still be incredibly sick with each treatment.

So, this week I decided that it must be a spiritual battle. I wasn't sure exactly how to fight this battle but pulled out a verse that I memorized many years ago.

"We demolish arguments and every pretension that sets itself up against the knowledge of God, and we take captive every thought to make it obedient to Christ." 2 Corinthians 10:5 (NIV)

I've never really been sure how to take my thoughts captive to Christ, but I thought it was worth a shot. First thing Monday morning, before I even got out of bed, I began to pray about my treatment this week; that it would accomplish what it was supposed to accomplish in my physical body - the destruction of any random cancer cells floating around - and I began to pray about the nausea issue. I just said out loud that I was taking every thought of nausea, every urge to gag, and anything related to it captive to Christ.

I didn't think much about it until Monday afternoon after having five hours of chemicals pumped into my body. Before I even left the doctor's office I was feeling sick, but with each wave of nausea I began repeating in my mind that I was taking that thought captive to Christ. The most amazing thing happened. Every single time I fought the nausea by repeating God's Word, it went away! I know that sounds weird, and I can't explain it except to say that His Word is powerful. I obviously need to tap into that power more in my life.

So, to anyone else out there struggling with your thought life, I encourage you to *"take captive every thought to make it obedient to Christ."* Like me, you may be surprised by the power He has given us.

Saturday January 2, 2010

I am slowly recovering from my last chemo treatment. I finished my home IV fluids today. I am feeling much better, just very weak. The weakness seems to last longer with each treatment, so I continue to concentrate on resting and trusting that God is in charge of my time schedule! "How weak?" you may ask... it took all my strength to open a can of biscuits this morning. Seriously. I had to sit down afterward! Two treatments to go!

"Be joyful in hope, patient in affliction, faithful in prayer." Romans 12:12 (NIV)

Tuesday January 5, 2010
His Purpose

The last chemo treatment really seemed to sap my energy. I have been resting and enjoying time with the girls while they are home. I had blood work done on Monday. My platelets were down to 34, which is pretty low. They need to be back up to at least 100 by next Monday so I can receive my next chemo treatment. That really would be a miracle for it to come up that high that fast. I am asking God for that miracle. I would really like to get these treatments done and be finished.

The nice thing for me with all this down time is that I have plenty of time to read, pray, study, and meditate on the things God is showing me. I also have had time to watch every college football bowl game that has been televised. How weird is that? I normally enjoy watching a few of my favorite teams play football, but I don't normally just watch games between teams that I am not interested in. This year has been different. Somehow it just seemed that I should be watching the games. The even stranger thing is God even used football to draw me closer to Him. Funny how He is always working and drawing us to Him if we will just take notice.

During one of the games one of the players had a Scripture reference on his cheekbones: John 17:17. I decided that I would look the verse up in my Bible and this is what it says:

"Sanctify them by the truth. Your word is truth." John 17:17 (NIV)

"Sanctify" is one of those churchy words that we don't hear or use often, and because of that I don't understand it very well. I decided to look up the definition of the word and this is what it said:

sanctification [san(k)-te-fe-eka-shen] *noun*
the process through which a person is incorporated ever more fully into the spiritual reality of Christ
given entirely to a specific person, activity, or cause
the active dedication of a thing to a single purpose.

God reminded me that in this new year I need to be actively dedicated to a single purpose. His purpose. That's sanctification. And John 17:17 says that the way to do that is by God's truth - His Word. I need to be so bathed in God's Word that it transforms me, it sanctifies me, it causes me to be actively dedicated to His purpose in my life.

I spent the afternoon praying. Thanking God for His reminder, even through a college bowl game, and asking Him to flood my life and my mind with His words; to invade my thoughts with His truth; to remind me to keep my Bible out and read it daily; to memorize it and put it into practice in my life.

That's my prayer for this New Year. I started the year cancer free! There is no better reason to spend the rest of the year praising Him, and letting Him sanctify me for His purpose!

Wednesday January 6, 2010
Meltdown

Today we had scheduled a meeting with some of the top staff leadership at the church. The plan was to pray and discuss our dreams and plans for the church for the New Year and beyond. I normally don't get out and do much of anything the week after my chemo treatments until the following weekend, saving up all my energy so that I can go to church that weekend. But today I really wanted to be a part of this meeting. I thought that if I could just get dressed and get there then I would be sitting most of the day. I should be able to do that, right?

Wrong. Most of the morning went well. I was so happy to actually be sitting in a room with some of my favorite people, praying together, sharing together what God has been teaching each of us, and seeking God's direction for our church. But then it hit me. We were walking to the building where they had our lunch prepared when my constant enemy – fatigue – took over. Ignoring the truth, I decided that I just needed to eat and then I would feel better. Of course what I really needed was to go home and keep resting.

Finally I realized that I had overdone things and headed out to the car. Before I was anywhere near the car I was short of breath, I could barely carry my purse (that, of course, may be due to other issues!), and I was hurting all over. I was completely exhausted. This is where meltdown #545 began.

The tears started and they didn't stop all the way home. I was so frustrated and angry. I don't want to be this person. I am so sick and tired of being sick and tired! It feels endless, even though I can see the light at the end of the tunnel. I want my life back. God, do You hear me? I don't want to do this anymore!

I arrived home, dragged myself into the house and collapsed

LAURA SHOOK

in tears. My sweet Sarah was there; we sat on the couch and cried and prayed together. Gradually the meltdown ran its course, and I remembered that God is here, He knows and understands, He will walk with me all the way, even when I have no strength and can't do the things I want to do. His way is better.

"For I know the plans I have for you," says the Lord, *"They are plans for good and not for disaster, to give you a future and a hope." Jeremiah* 29:11 *(NIV)*

Thursday January 7, 2010
How it Works

Recently I had the opportunity to talk to two people who had been diagnosed and were being treated for the exact same type of cancer that I have. They are a few months behind me in treatment and are following me along the same path.

I have another friend who is recovering from surgery to remove her colon and have a permanent ileostomy created. We are ostomates! She is home from the hospital and adjusting to her new life. One of the neatest things for me has been the opportunity to share with her my experience and tips for living with an ileostomy. Not something that I ever expected to be one of my life experiences, but something that I am very grateful for.

I am so happy to be able to share information, encouragement, experiences, feelings, and hope with others who are facing all the same challenges and struggles. God has taken a very difficult situation in my life and used it for good in someone else's life. And that's how it's supposed to work. The difficulties, struggles, and triumphs in our lives are not random. They have been allowed by a loving God and orchestrated to be used for His good purposes.

He allows us to suffer, to struggle, to stretch, to grow, to

192

learn, to change, and to overcome in order that we can tell our story with those He brings into our lives.

I pray that I will always live to tell my story – a story of God's goodness, His faithfulness, His truth, His strength, His kindness, and His love.

"Go home to your own (family and relatives and friends) and bring back word to them of how much the Lord has done for you, and (how He has) had sympathy for you and mercy on you." Mark 5:19 (AMP)

Friday January 8, 2010
Getting Ready

Newsflash: I put my boots on the right feet today.

The every-other-week schedule of chemotherapy has become routine now. I have learned that there are certain things that I need to make sure are done before I go back for chemotherapy on Monday. So, today I ventured out to the grocery store. It was a much more successful outing than my last one. It was very cold, so I bundled up with multiple gloves, boots, coat, and scarf. Isn't this Houston? Where did this cold come from? I did not feel quite as weak as I did the other day. I walked slowly through the store, depending on my cart to keep me upright. I purchased the necessities: dog food, cat food, cat litter, and food for the pantry so that Mark and Ashley will have something to eat next week. I made it home without a single tear.

Sunday January 10, 2010
I Will Not Forget You

I had a conversation with God yesterday about the fact that I really want to be able to have my chemotherapy treatment this week. I am so ready to be finished and to begin to regain my strength and my life. And then He reminded me that He is in control of my chemotherapy schedule.

It was such a stark reminder because each time it seems to be controlled by lab results and the oncologist's decision. I've been looking at it wrong again. God is in control. He always has been, even the weeks when treatment has been postponed. He is doing what is best for me. How easily I start to look at this world around me and forget that I am the daughter of the King of the Universe.

Again, Lord, I choose to trust You. I commit myself to You. I commit my treatment schedule to You. Thank You for doing what is best for me. And thank You for the gentle reminder of your faithfulness.

"But I trust in your unfailing love. I will rejoice because you have rescued me." Psalm 13:5 (NLT)

"I will not forget you. See, I have written your name on my hand." Isaiah 49:15-16 (NCV)

Did you read what that says? "I will not forget you." GOD will not forget me! The Holy God, creator of the universe, omnipotent, all powerful, all loving King of Kings and Lord of Lords will not forget ME! He will not forget any of us. I let that sink in.

Monday January 11, 2010
I Press On

I woke up this morning with a raised bruise on my right ankle. This is not necessarily surprising because I bruise easily and I am a klutz, but I thought that it might be a sign that my platelet count was not yet where it needed to be to have my chemo treatment today. Sure enough, when they did the lab work, my platelet count was still too low. No chemotherapy today.

I discussed a new issue with the nurses today. Apparently

I have eaten something that has caused problems with my digestive system. In spite of the long acting anti-diarrhea injection that I received last week, I have had diarrhea and massive amounts of gas since Wednesday night. Imodium is working to stop the diarrhea, I am faithfully drinking Pedialyte, but nothing has helped to get rid of the gas! This is especially fun with an ileostomy. I have to get up multiple times during the night to empty the bag, which swells up like a giant balloon. I'm honestly surprised it hasn't popped yet, which really would be fun!

They decided to test me for parasites and amoebas just to make sure that I haven't picked up something that is causing all this intestinal distress. Before I left the doctor's office they gave me a big plastic bag of supplies for collecting "specimens" to take to the lab. Can anything be more humiliating that carrying your own stool samples to the lab to drop them off?

So, I am back to waiting, resting, and trusting. Physically, I am very tired. Emotionally, I am very weary of the fight; and not just my struggle, but the struggle of so many special friends who are daily fighting for their lives. Spiritually, I press on, knowing that God is good and He has my name written on the palm of His hand.

Wednesday January 13, 2010
Out of These Ashes

The humiliating lab testing was worth it. I got results today. I have a bacterial infection called *Clostridium difficile*. This is a bacterium that normally resides in our intestines, but the chemotherapy has killed off most of the natural flora of my system, allowing these particular bacteria to grow out of control. This is usually a condition seen in hospital patients and nursing homes, and in people with weakened immune systems. It is a weird feeling to be diagnosed with an infection that normally strikes elderly, weakened nursing home residents. I am only forty-six.

As I contemplate my condition, I turn on Steve Curtis Chapman's CD "Beauty Will Rise," and I am overwhelmed with the lyrics.

"It was the day the world went wrong
I screamed till my voice was gone
And watched through the tears as everything
Came crashing down
Slowly panic turns to pain
As we awake to what remains
And sift through the ashes that are left behind
But buried deep beneath
All our broken dreams
We have this hope:
Out of these ashes... beauty will rise
And we will dance among the ruins
We will see Him with our own eyes
Out of these ashes... beauty will rise
For we know, joy is coming in the morning...
In the morning, beauty will rise
So take another breath for now,
And let the tears come washing down,
And if you can't believe I will believe
for you.
Cuz I have seen
the signs of spring!
Just watch and see:
Out of these ashes... beauty will rise
And we will dance among the ruins
We will see Him with our own eyes

Out of these ashes... beauty will rise
For we know, joy is coming in the morning...
In the morning..."

Today I choose to believe that out of these ashes beauty will rise.

Friday January 15, 2010
Waves of Grief

grief [gri:f] *noun*
deep or intense sorrow or distress
something that causes keen distress or suffering
something that causes great unhappiness
deep mental anguish

In the early days of my diagnosis I experienced a lot of vivid dreams in which I was grieving. These dreams have returned this week.

I had a hard time falling asleep the other night. I used that time to pray for all those I know who are also struggling with cancer. I finally fell asleep, only to wake myself up sobbing a couple of hours later.

I had been dreaming of a big party at our house. All of our friends were there. In my dream I had a collection of porcelain figurines and someone accidentally knocked them to the floor shattering them all. When I looked down at the floor, each piece of shattered porcelain had the face of someone I know who is fighting cancer, or has fought cancer. In my dream I began to cry uncontrollably, feeling such grief for these special friends. My grief woke me up and I found that I was sobbing in my bed, giant tears falling on my pillow, anguished for so many special people who are struggling against this nightmare disease. I finally realized that I had been dreaming and I was able to calm myself down.

Grief comes in waves. It comes unexpectedly. It comes at weird times. It even comes in dreams. It has been a constant companion all these months. But in the midst of the tears I have known the comfort only a father can give. The comfort of my Heavenly Father – protecting me, providing for me, flooding me with strength, peace, freedom, and hope. Thank You, God, for drying my tears in the night.

Monday January 18, 2010
And We Wait

My platelets are *still* too low to receive chemotherapy. They only came up from 71 to 75 over the course of the last week. I was so frustrated this morning. Not only because I am so ready to be finished with all of this, but also because it was another reminder of how sick I am. Healthy people don't have this problem. Only sick people. And I don't want to be reminded that I am still fighting a deadly disease.

Even my nurse was frustrated for me today. So frustrated that she cussed for me. She said that she knew I wouldn't, so she was doing it for me. I have the best nurses around!

So, we are back to waiting... again.

I know that God is doing what is best for me, but I am not a very good "waiter." I guess He knows this; and apparently it is a skill that He really wants me to learn.

"We wait in hope for the Lord; He is our help and our shield. In him our hearts rejoice, for we trust in his holy name." Psalm 33:20-21 (NIV)

"The Lord is my portion; therefore I will wait for him. The Lord is good to those whose hope is in him, to the one who seeks him; it is good to wait quietly for the salvation of the Lord." Lamentations 3:24-26 (NIV)

Tuesday January 19, 2010
Loyal Friends

"A friend is always loyal, and a brother is born to help in time of need."
Proverbs 17:17 (NLT)

I am constantly grateful for all my friends. Just when I think I can't go one more step...

A friend shows up with potato soup, with homemade bread, with waffles, with toilet paper, with a text message, with a Facebook message, with a timely comment, with an encouraging card, with a verse of Scripture, with a hand to hold, with a shoulder to cry on.

I couldn't do this without my friends. I know some friends feel helpless or feel that they haven't done enough to help us during this time. They will never know what they have truly done for us. The smallest kindnesses and the prayers are carrying us through, even when they don't realize it. I am eternally grateful for my friends.

Wednesday January 20, 2010
On a Positive Note

On the way home from the doctor's office on Monday I had to practice being positive. It takes practice for me. Here are a few of the good things I came up with.

1. I didn't feel sick when I walked in the house.
2. ....

Well, that's all I got! Like I said, I have to practice being positive.

But since then I have been able to see a few advantages to having an extra week off from chemotherapy.

1. I am able to go to our Ladies Bible Study this week. I am so

excited! I have missed my girls.

2. I actually ate frozen yogurt the other day. Being three weeks away from my last treatment, the nerves in my throat have calmed down. It still didn't taste right due to the constant metal taste in my mouth, but it was cold.

3. I had the strength to babysit a friend's precious little girl.

"For as he thinks within himself, so he is." Proverbs 23:7 (NAS)

Thursday January 21, 2010
Unbalanced

One of the funnier side effects of chemotherapy (maybe the only one?) is that my balance has been affected. If I close my eyes or pick up one foot I start to lean. I'm pretty sure no one else notices this but I sure feel it and it makes me laugh. I have wondered what would happen if I were pulled over by the police. I am sure they would think I am driving under the influence of something! "Officer, I swear, I haven't been drinking!"

The other day I accidentally got waterproof mascara on the end of my nose. Not just a little bit, but a big smear - several big spots. I tried to wipe it off, but because it was waterproof it wouldn't just wipe off. Naturally, I got distracted by something else and never removed the mascara from my nose. A little while later the doorbell rang. It was a couple of high school students selling pizza kits and cookie dough to raise money for their choir. Of course, I am a sucker for the kids out fundraising. I talked to the students for a few minutes, asking them all about their choir. They spent time telling me about the products they were selling and I placed my order. Then I gave them a business card from our church, told them my husband was the pastor, and invited them to come see us sometime. Later, I walked into the bathroom, looked in the mirror, and I was horrified! I just spent ten minutes talking to people at my door with mascara all over my nose. I even told them that Mark is the pastor of the church! I can just imagine them walking away and discussing my appearance. I guess I am unbalanced in more ways than one.

Saturday January 23, 2010
Perfect Faithfulness

The song in my head all week has been one of Christy Nockels new songs, "Healing is in Your Hands." The lyrics are beautiful:
> "No mountain, no valley, no gain or loss we know
> could keep us from Your love
> No sickness, no secret, no chain is strong enough
> to keep us from Your love
> to keep us from Your love
> How high, how wide
> No matter where I am, healing is in Your hands
> How deep, How strong,
> And now by Your grace I stand, healing is in Your hands"

As those lyrics played in my head, I read this verse in my Bible: *"O Lord, You are my God; I will exalt You, I will give thanks to Your name; for You have worked wonders, plans formed long ago, with perfect faithfulness." Isaiah 25:1 (NAS)*

I sit here this morning contemplating those things. I just read an update from a friend who has been in and out of the hospital this week, trying to figure out the source of the deep and constant pain in her lower back and leg. Yesterday, after hours of testing and waiting, they heard the results that they suspected. Her cancer has returned, invading her bones.

Waves of grief and anger wash over me. I wish I could do this for her. I wish I could take away her pain. And then God reminds me that *He* is doing it for her. Just like He planned my life, He planned my friend's life long ago, with *perfect faithfulness*. He is with her. He feels her pain. He hears her cries. He holds her tears in His hands. He is faithful. He is good. Even when I don't understand. Even when I can't see it.

The song lyrics come back to my head: *"Our present, our future, our past is in your hands… And now by your grace I stand, healing is in your hands."*

Sunday January 24, 2010
Follow Me

On the coffee table is a magazine with a famous actor pictured on the front and the words, "Follow me." Of course, he is asking people to follow him on Twitter. Due to the fact that I am technically challenged, I don't have a Twitter account or follow anyone on Twitter, but it is interesting to see this phenomenon sweep across our country - people connecting by "following."

This reminds me of a story from the Bible found in the book of John. Jesus is talking to Peter and He foretells how life will be for him leading up to his death. He tells Peter that he won't be able to dress himself, or feed himself, he won't be able to see. Essentially, He tells Peter that life is going to be hard, and then you die. I can imagine Peter thinking, "Wow, Jesus, thanks for that." But then Jesus says something interesting. He says to Peter, "Follow Me." Your life is going to be difficult. That's the truth. That's just the way it is. So follow Me.

God whispers to me, that's what I want you to know too. This may be a great year, or it may be a really difficult year with unwelcome surprises, unexpected interruptions, heartache or tragedy – and just like He said to Peter, Jesus says to me, "Follow

Me." That's the only way to make it through life. I have to follow Him.

In my journey through cancer I don't know the future. I don't know what's coming around the bend. I haven't been able to make any plans because I don't know from one week to the next what my schedule will be. My life is totally in the hands of God - His plans, His timing, His long-term goals. I can't see any of it. And the things I can see are scary.

Learning to follow has been a process filled with multiple conversations like this one:

Laura: "I am all by myself."

God: "Follow Me. I am with you."

Laura: "I am scared."

God: " Follow Me. I will take care of you."

Laura: "I don't like this."

God: "Follow Me. I am working for your good."

Laura: "I can't see where I'm going."

God: "Follow Me. I know the way."

Laura: " I can't see the path."

God: "Follow Me. Don't follow the path."

Follow Me. *Follow Me.* **Follow Me**. That is His instruction for us. Jesus was the first one to ask people to follow Him all those years ago as He called His disciples. And today He calls us too, to follow Him and connect with Him.

"Then Jesus told him, 'Follow me.'" John 21:19 (NLT)

Monday January 25, 2010
Return of the Platelets

My platelets jumped from 75 to 185 over the last week! So, I started chemo round seven today. It seemed weird this week to pray for platelets and to pray to be able to have chemo – in essence praying that I would be able to be sick all week. But, it feels really good to know that after this week I only have one more treatment to go!

All the usual side effects are back. The doctor said that my equilibrium issues are most likely due to one of the drugs I'm receiving. He told me to be careful of policemen and to make sure that they give me a breath test if they stop me. Thankfully, it doesn't really effect my driving.

Friday January 29, 2010
Hello World

I have been sleeping about twenty hours a day for the past four days. I didn't know that was humanly possible, but it is. It's Friday morning and I feel like I am Sleeping Beauty waking from a deep sleep. Sadly, there was no handsome prince involved, and at this point I probably more closely resemble a hibernating bear or frog. That could explain the missing prince! Honestly, the "prince" has been sleeping a lot as well. The endurance marathon called cancer seems to sap everyone's energy.

This round of chemo has seemed a little easier. Thankfully I have not been quite as sick to my stomach this time. I am still extremely weak, and I still hurt all over, but things are beginning to turn around.

The best part is knowing that I only have one more round to go. I try to get excited about that, and I am, but I have experienced so many surprises in the past eight months that I don't want to get too excited yet. I don't really know what the doctor will say when we are finished. I don't know what the follow-up treatment will involve. I don't know how quickly my strength and energy will return to normal levels. And I do know that I still have another surgery to go. So for now I am cautiously optimistic that we are nearing the end of this part of the journey.

Wednesday February 3, 2010
Safe in Your Arms

Yesterday turned out to be an emotional day for me. I'm not sure why. Mark says it must be post-traumatic stress. Lots of emotions have been tucked away as our attention has been focused on fighting this battle. Now, with this part of the journey winding down and the end in sight, it is safe to let some of the emotions come to the surface. All those emotions spilled over into my dreams again.

All night I dreamed that I was being chased. Something unseen and deadly was coming after me. I was in fear for my life. Adrenaline would shoot through my system and I would wake up, heart pounding, only to find myself safe in my bed. They were only dreams. The truth is that no one was chasing me, I was safe.

I woke up this morning with God whispering in my heart, "The same is true in your life, Laura. No matter how you feel, keep your eyes on My truth. Take your thoughts captive to Christ. You are safe in My arms."

This is one of my favorite aspects of God's character. He is big enough, strong enough, caring enough to keep me safe.

"But as for me, I will sing about your power. Each morning I will sing with joy about your unfailing love. For you have been my refuge, a place of safety when I am in distress." Psalm 59:16 (NLT)

"During danger he will keep me safe in his shelter. He will hide me in his Holy Tent, or he will keep me safe on a high mountain." Psalm 27:5 (NCV)

Friday February 5, 2010
What If I Asked

Mark and I served as missionaries in Mexico City for almost eight years. I first began dreaming of being a missionary when I was seventeen. Fourteen years later we sold everything we owned, Mark quit his job, we uprooted our kids, moved away from our family, our friends, and our church and went for our dream. It was an amazing time in our lives. God taught us so many lessons, we made some of the most amazing friends, and we fell in love with the people of Latin America.

In 2003 I remember sitting alone one day, asking God for wisdom and direction for our lives, when I quietly heard Him whisper, "What if I ask you to give it all up and go back to the United States?"

My response to Him went like this, "But I already did that! We already gave it all up. We sold our house, our cars, everything we owned, left Mark's job, and our families. We already did that, God."

And again He softly spoke, "What if I asked you to do it all again? Give up *your* dream and step out into My dream for you again?"

I struggled with my thoughts, my feelings, and my faith for a little while. Then I quietly answered, "Well I guess I'd do it again."

And so we returned to Houston with no plans and no jobs, just a sure trust that God knew what He was doing.

Fast-forward to 2009. I am diagnosed with cancer and it just so happens that I live in one of the best cities in the world for cancer research and treatment. God knew what He was doing.

I am living in the same city as my parents, my brother, and my in-laws who have been an amazing support to me this past year. God knew what He was doing.

I am surrounded by the best friends ever, who have cheered me on, listened to me, cried with me, laughed with me, and not let anything fall through the cracks! God knew what He was doing.

I am part of the most incredible church family on the planet! Just last night at our worship and prayer service, I was surrounded by a giant group of the most awesome people who laid their hands on me and prayed for me again, and told me over and over that they pray for me daily. God knew what He was doing.

God, may I always choose to go with Your dreams. You can see around the corner, You know what the future holds. You know what You are doing.

"Take delight in the Lord, and he will give you your heart's desires. Commit everything you do to the Lord. Trust him, and he will help you." *Psalm 37:4-5 (NLT)*

Saturday February 6, 2010
No Taste

Sad day. One of my favorite things is Brach's candy corn. I usually only buy it around Halloween, but I bought a bag the other day and brought it home. I opened the bag today, looking forward to enjoying the sweet little candies, and guess what? I couldn't taste them at all! Not at all. Zero taste. Nothing. The chemo drugs have erased my ability to enjoy candy corn (and most other foods!) by wiping out my taste buds.

I'm not sure why I thought I would be able to taste the candy. My sense of taste has been missing from the beginning of my treatment. Most foods now have a metallic taste. This combined with nausea and no appetite make eating very difficult. Just like every other cancer patient, I am struggling to keep weight on my body. I see now how cancer causes a body to waste away. I have determined to make myself eat something every two hours, no matter what it is, just to get calories in my body. Mark does a great job of buying anything that sounds remotely appetizing to me, but I struggle to eat nonetheless. Thankfully, this side effect should be temporary, improving when I am finally finished pumping these drugs into my body. Here's hoping.

Monday February 8, 2010
Be Sure of This

Cancer can be lonely.

I have so many beautiful people around me walking this journey with me and yet much of the time I feel very alone. I think one of the hardest things is that even the people who I am closest to can't really understand how it feels. We are not able to relate in that way because they haven't been down the same road exactly. They can sympathize, and listen, and care, and provide for me, but they can't know how it feels. It's no one's fault. That's just how it is. Unless you have been diagnosed with cancer yourself, you just can't know completely how it feels.

I can't understand completely how my closest family and friends feel either. I haven't been in their shoes as a family member of a cancer patient. So there is a disconnect that manifests itself in loneliness.

I know that God wants to use this feeling to teach me more about who He is. And to teach me that I am totally dependent on Him and no one else, even when I think I can handle things myself. It is always about God and me. Will I trust that He's here even in the loneliest moments? Will I wait for Him and listen for Him? Will I run to Him?

When my children were little (and still to this day) whenever they were feeling lonely, or afraid, or facing new challenges, I would tell them to remember that they are never alone. Jesus is always walking with them. I would tell them in those frightening moments to squeeze their hand and remember who is holding it.

I am squeezing my hand today. Thank You, God, that You are here.

"And be sure of this: I am with you always..." Matthew 28:20 (NLT)

"Though they stumble, they will never fall, for the Lord holds them by the hand." Psalm 37:24 (NLT)

Tuesday February 9, 2010
I'm Longing

I had an appointment with the oncologist yesterday. My platelets were up to 88, a good jump, but not high enough to get that last chemo treatment. I wasn't really surprised and so I wasn't really disappointed. One thing I have definitely learned in the last eight months is that God is completely in charge of my treatment schedule, and He knows what He's doing. So, I'll enjoy my week off and get ready to be sick next week.

We did have the opportunity to discuss what my follow-up care will look like. It seemed sort of surreal to actually be talking about the weeks and months (and years!) *after* I am finished with all my cancer treatment. It was exciting to think that I will actually be finished with all of this and to know that day is coming up soon. And, knowing my love for planning and schedules, it was exciting to be able to see that there will be a pretty routine schedule. Wow, I might actually get my life back!

I will have a PET scan two weeks after my last chemo treatment. I will have surgery to close the ileostomy six weeks after my last chemo treatment. Then going forward I will have a PET scan or CT scan (depending on what the insurance company will approve) every three months the first year following treatment, every four months the second year, every six months the third year, and then if everything looks good I will have one annually after that. Of course there will be annual colonoscopies thrown in just for fun! So, I am still going to be pretty close to my oncologist and his staff.

The frequent scans are to try to catch any recurrence early if it happens. That is a good thing. But it also messes with my mind a little.

I truly believe that God has healed me of cancer. I truly believe that I will grow old with Mark. But I wonder how I will deal with the thoughts and emotions related to frequent visits to the oncologist's office. How will I move forward with so many reminders of cancer? I don't really feel afraid of recurrence, but I feel afraid of feeling afraid.

Wednesday February 10, 2010
Lesson Learned

The challenge I see now is to go on living while holding on to all the things I've learned and incorporating them into my daily life. The habits I have been practicing during the last nine months are the habits I want to keep.

Choose to take every thought captive to Christ.

Choose to recognize His presence here with me.

Choose to recognize His sovereignty over my life.

Choose to trust in His plans.

Choose to leave my burdens with Him and take up His peace.

Choose to release control to the One who knows my future.

Choose to bathe my mind with His Words.

Choose to believe that He is good.

Choose to believe in His faithfulness.

Choose to praise Him.

Daily choices form daily habits. I'm glad He is helping me to make those choices. Lord, please continue to remind me of the lessons learned, and please keep teaching me. I want more of You.

Monday February 15, 2010
For My Good

Dear Bone Marrow,

I only have eleven ileostomy bags left. Please get yourself together and produce some platelets so I can have that last chemo treatment and surgery before I have to buy more bags. Thank you.

Sincerely,

Laura

I woke up today with the lyrics from one of the songs we sang at church this weekend playing over and over in my head: "You make all things work together for my good." I was looking forward to starting my last chemotherapy treatment today, and these lyrics reminded me to trust completely. Mark and I drove to the oncologist's office with perfect peace in our hearts.

Big Sigh. Unfortunately my platelets were still too low to receive chemotherapy this week. They did jump up from last week – all the way from 88 to 89! Again, we wait. Honestly, I am OK with waiting. I think everyone around me is more disappointed than I am. If I have learned anything over the last nine months it is that God works on His timetable and not mine.

After seeing the doctor I spent the next hour rescheduling chemo appointments, doctor's appointments, lab tests, and the PET scan. I'm sure they are probably all tired of hearing me call and say, "I need to reschedule my appointment, again."

If I actually receive chemo next week then I will finish my last treatment on Ashley's 19th birthday. What a nice birthday present for her and for me!

Wednesday February 17, 2010
Six-Pack Abs

I survived another appointment with the surgeon today. Quick probe of sights unseen prove that all has continued to heal well. The surgeon expects that I will have no problems when everything is put back into service again. If I start my last chemo treatment next week then I will have surgery to close the ileostomy the first week of April, assuming that all my blood counts are back up to normal levels at that time.

I did ask the doctor if he could restore my six-pack abs when he performs surgery. He laughed and said he will give me mine back just as soon as he gets his back!

Mark scheduled his colonoscopy today. He and my dad plan to have them done on the same day, a special family bonding moment! I am proud of these guys for getting it done. Early detection is the key. Thank you, Mark and Daddy! I love you both!

Sunday February 21, 2010
Glimpse of Heaven

Mark and I were hanging out together on Friday night, talking about life and what's to come. As I shared with Mark I began to cry again - hoping that I would have the chance to live out my dreams - dreams of a long life with Mark, time spent with my favorite people in my favorite places, and sharing the love of Christ around the world. They seemed like pretty good dreams to me.

But even as I poured my heart out to Mark, God opened up my eyes to see even greater things. He gave me a tiny glimpse of Heaven. He reminded me that Mark and I have eternity together. Forever together! And as nice as my dreams may seem, God has planned things I can't even imagine. I dream of eighty or more years with Mark and time spent in Latin America and Africa. He dreams of eternity with Mark and travel to unimaginable places with God-sized jobs to do. Wow! How small my dreams seem in comparison to His!

God, count me in. I want Your dreams.

"Trust God from the bottom of your heart; don't try to figure out everything on your own. Listen for God's voice in everything you do, everywhere you go; he's the one who will keep you on track." Proverbs 3:5-6 *(The Message)*

Monday February 22, 2010
Last Chemo Treatment

Today I woke up with Kim Walker's "How He Loves Us" playing over and over in my head:

"He is jealous for me. Love's like a hurricane,
I am a tree bending beneath the weight of
His wind and mercy
When all of a sudden, I am unaware of these afflictions eclipsed by glory
and I realize just how beautiful you are and how great
your affections are for me.

Oh, how He loves us so
Oh, how He loves us
How He loves us so.
Yeah, He loves us

Oh, how He loves us
Oh, how He loves us
Oh, how He loves."

I am excited, hoping that I will be able to begin my last chemo treatment today. We arrive at the doctor's office, have blood drawn and wait for the results. The nurse comes and tells us that my platelet count is 145. Then she says, "But your white blood cell count is low, I'm going to go show it to the doctor."

"No!" I think to myself. God, please don't let my white cells keep me from getting treatment today.

The nurse returns and gives me the thumbs-up sign. Finally! I feel like sobbing, but stifle my tears, knowing if I start crying I'll never stop.

Tuesday February 23, 2010
Sick

I wake up and wish I didn't have to get out of bed. I really think they should come to my house to give me today's infusion.
I roll out of bed and the minute my feet hit the ground I am vomiting. This continues all day, every time I move, in spite of all the nausea medications I have taken. I guess I am going to finish with a bang.

Not a fun day, but *tomorrow* I will receive the last of the drugs and *ring the bell*! I am so thrilled that I will be finished with this part of my treatment.

Wednesday February 24, 2010
Ring That Bell!

Wednesday morning I wake up knowing this is the day I will ring the bell signifying the end of my chemotherapy treatments. After so many months and delays it hardly seems real. I get out of bed, thankful my stomach has calmed down since Tuesday.

At 7:30 a.m. my 48-hour IV pump beeps that it is empty. I start crying and can hardly hold myself up. That beep signals the end of the toxic chemicals. The last drop has entered my blood stream to do its job. I'm done! I did it! I survived IV chemotherapy! This was the part that I most dreaded about cancer treatment and honestly I didn't think that I would be able to make it through. Together with God's strength and the love and support of my family and friends, I have done it!

Mark and I arrive at the oncologist's office at 9:15 a.m. and are soon followed by my parents and nearly the whole Community of Faith staff. They have all come to witness the bell ringing and to celebrate with me. My heart is so full I am speechless! All the nurses, lab technicians, pharmacists, medical assistants, receptionists, and my doctors dropped what they were doing and came to watch me ring the bell. There were so many cameras it felt like the paparazzi were there!

I looked up at that bell, read the plaque above it, "Believe in miracles," and I rang that bell for the whole world to know - God did this! He is good. He has walked with me every step. I do believe in miracles!

I hope my friends around the world heard it ringing! That was my intention!

"The Lord has saved us! Let's celebrate! We waited and hoped — now our God is here." Isaiah 25:9 (CEV)

Friday February 26, 2010
Wait and Rest

Everyone wants to know how I feel now that I've finished chemotherapy. I'm sure they are wondering how I feel emotionally, but all I can feel right now is how I am physically - just like after every other treatment. I have slept most of this week, day and night, I have been sick at my stomach, and I am very, very weak. But each day is a little better than the last.

I have had food cravings for corn bread and chicken fried steak; and thankfully I have an awesome husband and friends who go the distance to make those dreams come true. I'm just glad I feel like eating anything at all.

My one wish now is for a time machine so that I could move on into next week and feel good.

God's Spirit whispers again, "Wait. Rest. Wait. Rest."
And so I do.

Saturday February 27, 2010
The Girls are Back in Town!

Friday night Mark and I were watching the winter Olympics, hoping that the U.S. would come through for us in speed skating. At 9:30 p.m. the doorbell rang. We both looked at each other, but neither of us was expecting anyone. Because I had not properly bathed since the start of chemo on Monday, Mark had the job of answering the door.

As soon as he opened the door we was bombarded with cheering, party horns, balloons and hats accompanied by three smiling faces! Our daughters, Sarah and Ashley had driven down from Oklahoma, picked up their sweet friend Callie, and come home to celebrate the end of chemotherapy with their mom. What a special surprise! I have the sweetest girls in the world!

Tuesday March 2, 2010
New Week

Usually the week following chemotherapy I continue resting and gradually begin to get all the things done that didn't get done the week before. This week has been the same except for one twist. I know that I am finished with chemotherapy!

Monday I went to have blood work done, as usual. My platelets have dropped down to forty-three and my white cell count has dropped. Both of those things were expected following my treatment. A platelet count of forty-three is hovering just over a dangerous level, so I was given specific instructions to watch for bruising and bleeding of any kind and to call the doctor if that happens. I've been in this position before, so I don't expect there to be any problems. I will have my blood checked again next Monday just to make sure that the platelet level has begun to climb and not continued to decrease.

I have to tell you that it felt really good to walk into the oncologist's office knowing that I would not be receiving any more chemotherapy. I think I was walking taller and I certainly had a bigger smile on my face!

Wednesday March 3, 2010
Pleasures of the Day

"You will show me the way of life, granting me the joy of your presence and the pleasure of living with you forever." Psalm 16:11 (NLT)

Psalm 16 is one of my favorites. As I was reading it this morning I was keenly aware of God's presence, His joy, and His pleasures in my life. Now that I have finished my chemo treatments and am beginning to get my strength back, every day seems full of possibility and promise!

Here are a few of my pleasures of the day:
- Waking up after a full night's sleep.
- Driving to somewhere other than a doctor's office.
- Cleaning the kitchen without getting tired.
- Planning my parents 50th Anniversary Party.
- Getting back to work.
- Sunshine and sixty-two degrees.
- Receiving good news from a sweet friend.

Sunday March 7, 2010
I Know

One of my favorite songs is "You Are For Me" by Kari Jobe. It is one of the songs that frequently plays in my head and heart, and it has helped carry me through the past nine months.

This weekend it was one of the songs we sang at Community of Faith. One of our worship leaders, Robin, sang the song as we all shared communion together. Robin has a beautiful voice and it is easy to just sit back, close your eyes, and feel God's love wash over you as she sings the words of this song.

But for me, I can't help but be on my feet belting out the words of this song with a huge smile on my face! Over and over in the song we sang out the words, "I know." These words seem so simple, but after all I have experienced and faced since last May, they are the most incredible words to me. *I know.* I have learned so much about the character, goodness, faithfulness, strength, peace, and truth of my God that singing those words produces a wellspring of gratitude and joy in me that can't help but come out.

I know *God!* I *know* Him. Like I never have before. We have such an intimacy now that makes me want to know Him more. And it also makes me feel sorry for those who don't know

Him. He *is* life. No matter what happens, as I travel this path through cancer and follow-up care, I am OK. I've seen God; I've experienced His Holiness. I know. And nothing can shake that.

"Let all that I am wait quietly before God, for my hope is in him. He alone is my rock and my salvation, my fortress where I will not be shaken." Psalm 62:5-6 (NLT)

Tuesday March 9, 2010
Nothing Is Impossible

In 1995 Mark and I moved to Costa Rica with our children to attend Spanish language school. We lived in a small house in the neighborhood surrounding the school. Most of the homes in Costa Rica are surrounded by walls, gates, and bars. It actually took four keys to get all the way into the front door of our house. The back yard was surrounded by a concrete block wall that was at least eight feet tall. Nothing was going to get in or out of that house that wasn't supposed to!

One of the most amazing things about Costa Rica was the beautiful scenery. The rich volcanic soil and abundance of annual rainfall produced beautiful vegetation. The fence posts would actually sprout and grow during the rainy season.

I remember one day feeling overwhelmed with the stress of moving to a new country, living in a new culture, and learning a new language. I was struggling to see my way through, and wondering if we had made the right decision in going there. I walked out into the backyard, thinking, and praying, and much to my surprise I found a beautiful flower growing out of the concrete wall. It was in full bloom. It was the most incredible sight! How was that possible?

In that moment, God reminded me that nothing was impossible for Him. It gave me hope and courage to continue.

"For nothing is impossible with God." Luke 1:37 (NLT)

This week I was reminded again. I walked out the front door the other day to find a single red rose blooming, and God whispered in my ear, "Remember the lesson of the flower in the wall in Costa Rica? It's still true. Nothing is impossible for Me."

I am trusting God to continue to do the impossible.

Tuesday March 11, 2010
Today I Am Scared

My next PET scan is scheduled for Wednesday, March 17th. I haven't had one since the original scan in June of last year. And I haven't been worried about it at all. In fact I was so calm about it that I began to worry that I wasn't worried. (I have to have SOMETHING to worry about, right?) I really believe that God has healed me, so certainly the scan will show that.

Then today comes. And I am scared. My mind starts to play games. All the things I have learned about rectal cancer begin to play in my head. Rectal cancer has a high recurrence rate, and it most often recurs close to the original site or in the organs of the pelvic region. My thoughts are totally fabricated, and they spiral, totally out of control. Fear takes over, an unwelcome enemy.

Thankfully, the lessons I've learned begin to come into play: God is in control; God is in the future; take every thought captive to the obedience of Christ; focus on the truth; focus on today; reject lies; be clothed for battle, this is a war; pray continually; choose to trust; God *is* good.

Peace comes in like a wave washing over me. Thank You, God. I am yours.

"Hide me in the shadow of your wings." Psalm 17:8 (NLT)

Friday March 12, 2010
Cancer Humor

I got a letter in the mail today from an insurance company trying to sell me life insurance. I laughed out loud. What are the chances that someone would actually sell me life insurance now? Slim to none!

"He will once again fill your mouth with laughter and your lips with shouts of joy." Job 8:21 (NLT)

Monday March 15, 2010
God Celebrates Too

It's Monday morning, and for the first time in many months I do not have a doctor's appointment on Monday morning. It feels really strange. What do I do? I feel like God has given me back a tiny piece of my calendar.

Then I remember Mark's sermon yesterday about practicing the presence of Christ in our lives. I decide that if God is going to trust me with a tiny piece of the calendar, then I sure better include Him in my plans. I spend time with Him, praying, reading His Word, meditating, asking Him to help me be aware of His presence today.

He speaks His words to me in Zephaniah 3:17, *"The Lord your God wins victory after victory and is always with you. He celebrates and sings because of you, and He will refresh your life with His love." (CEV)*

What an amazing picture. God celebrates and sings because of me. Wow! How can that be? The perfect picture of a love relationship - each one celebrating and singing because of the other!

His praise plays in my heart and head the rest of the day.

"Praise belongs to you
Let every kingdom bow

Let every ocean roar
Let every heart adore you now

Praise belongs to you
What can I do but sing
The greatest joy I've found
Is to lay a crown before my King
Before my King"
("Glorified," by Jared Anderson)

Wednesday March 17, 2010
PET Scan

Today I had my first post-treatment PET/CT scan. The PET/CT scan is more accurate than a PET scan or CT scan alone. The two scans are put together to form a more complete picture of what is going on inside of the body. I am thankful that this is the scan my oncologist chose to have done.

I woke up this morning with praise music playing in my heart and in my head. It was there every time I woke up during the night last night. I did not feel nervous or worried at all. Mark and I actually made it to the appointment on time, which is very unusual for us.

The same man who performed my original PET scan last summer was there to greet me today. He let me take pictures of the lead lined equipment. They tested my blood glucose level (it was normal) and then injected me with a radioactive glucose solution. I spent the next hour in a small dark room resting and giving my body time to absorb the radioactive solution. I was then led into the room with the scanning equipment. I was positioned and strapped onto a narrow table with my hands over my head. The technician left me alone in the room.

For thirty minutes I was moved in and out of the scanning

machine. I was very careful to be still, but after several minutes in a cold room, even with a warm blanket, my muscles start to twitch, my mind starts to inch toward worry. I recognize the drift and begin to repeat Scripture and sing praise songs in my mind. I pray repeatedly that the scan will show that God has healed me, but I also pray that if there is anything the doctors need to see that this scan will show it to us.

When I am finished they give me a little gift bag including snacks. I am starved and dive in. They tell us that the radiologist will read the scan this afternoon and that my oncologist should have the results sometime Thursday or early Friday. I make a mental note of when to start calling the oncologist if they haven't called me first.

Mark and I drive home, where I fall asleep on the couch for two hours. I guess I was more stressed than I thought I was. I kind of want to just sleep until I get the results. Tears come. I am ready to know if I can go on living, or if I will have to continue fighting this disease.

Thursday March 18, 2010
While I'm Waiting

No news today. Still waiting. I did get a lot of phone calls today, but they weren't from the doctor. They were from Mark and my dad who are anxiously awaiting good news from the PET scan.

I am hoping that the doctor will call me with the results some time Friday.

John Waller's song, "While I'm Waiting," has played in my head all day:

"I'm waiting
I'm waiting on You, Lord
And I am hopeful

I'm waiting on You, Lord
Though it is painful
But patiently, I will wait

I will move ahead, bold and confident
Taking every step in obedience
While I'm waiting
I will serve You
While I'm waiting
I will worship
While I'm waiting
I will not faint
I'll be running the race
Even while I wait"

Friday March 19, 2010
Speechless

"No tumors were found. Your PET scan was normal."

Two simple sentences, and yet they left me speechless. I had hoped it was true, I had believed it was true, but to hear the actual words blew my mind! I felt as if my heart actually stopped for a split second. As surreal as it was to hear the words, "You have cancer," last May, it was just as mind boggling today to hear that there is no sign of the disease in my body. I feel like I am in shock again. I lie on the floor and breathe deep. I am alive. I am still alive! I get to go on living.

Thank You, Jesus, for hearing my prayers, and the prayers of so many others. Thank You that You are good, and that You would have still been good even if the results had been different. I love You!

Then I call Mark, and my parents, and frantically send text messages to everyone who was waiting with me. What an amazing group of family and friends. God has surrounded me with so much love and support.

My brother, Cary, responds to the text message with these words: "The PET scan may be normal, but that doesn't mean YOU are normal." I love that he always makes me laugh.

My friend Debbie calls from California, laughing, crying, and dancing. Then she says to me, "Welcome to the CANCER-FREE CLUB!"

I am cancer free!! I survived!! Thank You, Jesus!

"I will answer them before they even call to me. While they are still talking about their needs, I will go ahead and answer their prayers!" Isaiah 65:24 (NLT)

RECOVERY

"Hope cannot be destroyed.
It calls us to rise up; it whispers our name.
It draws us to believe that, sometimes,
wishes do come true."

Kim Meeder

Sunday March 21, 2010
Everything Is Yours

I have always loved music; especially music that expresses what is in my heart. For some reason, music touches my soul; it produces a strong connection between God and me. He often uses music to calm me, to teach me, to remind me, and to encourage me. And in some feeble way, I hope that my singing praise to Him lets Him know how much I love Him.

All through the months, there have been lyrics and music that have carried me through. Often they have produced tears. At times I have been so overwhelmed with God's goodness that I couldn't even sing. There have been times when I've felt that my chest would explode with the joy I have felt through the awareness of God with me and His peace and power in my life.

I'll never understand the enormity of God's love for me, or even why He would choose to love me, but He has given me tiny glimpses of that love through this journey. There are no words to tell Him how much I love Him and how grateful I am.

This weekend we sang a new song at church. It is based on a prayer of King David found in 2 Chronicles. How cool to know that I am singing words that King David penned so many years ago. Maybe one day we'll all sit down and sing it together with him at the feet of Jesus!

"We who are thirsty, we who are poor cry out to you
You have redeemed us by your mercy
We who are ransomed, we who are healed give honor to you
You have restored us with your blessing"
("Everything is Yours," by Amos Rivera and Donald Butler)

As we began to sing the words "We who are healed," Sarah leaned over and said, "That's you, mom." And my heart almost burst. That *is* me. I am healed.

God, I do give honor to You. You have restored me with Your blessing. I have no words to thank You enough. Everything in heaven and earth is Yours. I am Yours. Thank You.

Thursday March 25, 2010
Freedom

I had an appointment with the oncologist on Monday. He affirmed that my PET scan looked great. The whole office staff was so happy for me, smiling, hugging me, and congratulating me. He told me that I don't have to come see him again for three months. That feels really weird after making weekly (sometimes 3 times a week!) visits to his office since June. What will I do with all my free time?

My blood levels were all at nearly normal levels. He told me that I can go forward with surgery on April 6th to remove my port and close the ileostomy. He also told me that I could be in the sun now, just in time for summer. Can it really be true? Can I be getting my life back?

I saw the surgeon on Monday and he agreed that my PET scan looked really good. We discussed the surgery and what to expect as I recover. He said he would see me in a couple of weeks at the hospital.

Things I can do now:
1. Walk upstairs without getting tired
2. Drink cold water
3. Carry my purse
4. Clean the kitchen without getting tired
5. Eat ice cream

My energy is coming back and my taste buds are starting to come back. I still have some issues with the nerves in my fingertips and my feet, but that may take months to resolve.

Little by little, life goes on.

Sunday April 4, 2010
Keep On

The past six weeks since my last chemo treatment have been interesting for me. With the end of treatment and the good report from my PET scan everyone is very happy for me and excited to see how God has answered so many prayers. Lots of smiles, lots of hugs, lots of celebrating.

And then there's me. Somehow I'm just not quite able to completely celebrate. Don't get me wrong; I am so grateful for what God has done. But it is hard for my brain to wrap around the idea that this ordeal is really over. Ninety-nine percent of my brain is celebrating, but that nagging one percent keeps flashing warning signs. Don't get too happy. Don't celebrate too much. It could come back. You won't be considered healed until you've had five years of clear PET scans.

These thoughts stop me in my tracks. What do I do now? How do I move forward? How do I go on with my life without living in fear? And what exactly should my next steps be? Part of me thinks I should spend the next period of time getting ready – just in case – cleaning out the closets, getting rid of the clutter, organizing paperwork. The one percent tells me that I better get things in place while I'm healthy and feeling strong. Just in case. But the ninety-nine percent screams, "I don't want to live like that! I don't want to live in fear." How do I put those two thoughts together? How do I prudently get ready, just in case, while at the same time move forward with faith and trust?

Those have been my thoughts over these weeks, and my prayers. God, please show me how to move forward without fear. Show me what to do now.

Over the last few days, God has begun to answer my prayer. I read the same thing in several different places. That's always a sign to me that God wants me to hear something. Keep on. It's that simple. If I want to move forward without fear, I just keep on.

"Study My words and carry them out unflinchingly, unflinchingly." (*God Calling*)

"Jesus told the people who had faith in Him, 'If you keep on obeying what I have said, you truly are my disciples. You will know the truth and the truth will set you free.' " John 8:31-32 *(CEV)*

That's it. Continue to walk in obedience. Studying His words, putting them into practice in my life. That's the secret to moving forward and living without fear.

Monday April 5, 2010
Surgery, Round Three

Tuesday morning we will head back to the hospital for one more surgery. I will have my ileostomy closed and my intestinal system put back in working order. I will also be having my port removed from my chest. The surgery shouldn't take long, about an hour, but I will be in the hospital for three to four days. Surgery is scheduled for noon.

Goodbye ileostomy bag and hello Chili's Southwestern eggrolls!

Thursday April 8, 2010
Movement

When I worked as a nurse I worked mostly with elderly people. One of the daily topics of conversation was their bowel habits. I always thought it was funny, this fascination with constipation and regularity. And I thought it was especially funny that they always wanted to discuss it.

Well, now I totally understand! I'm sure this is more information than you ever wanted to know, and it probably shouldn't be published, but here goes.

I had a bowel movement this morning! Yes! My colon is awake and functioning after two surgeries, radiation, chemotherapy and eight months of rest. Isn't that amazing? Our bodies are "beautifully and wonderfully made," just like Scripture tells us.

I had my first regular meal last night. I don't think I'll ever eat Jell-O again.

The surgeon just came by to see me and he said I can go home today. Humpty Dumpty is back together again!

Friday April 9, 2010
I'll Stay Home

Thursday evening. Forty-eight hours post-op. Welcome back, my old friend - diarrhea.

Yes, one of the expected steps of recovery from my ileostomy reversal surgery is a period of time where my colon is relearning to do its job. Diarrhea has been a common theme as I've dealt with radiation and IV chemotherapy. Unfortunately, this time, I am not able to take any medication to stop the flow. We don't want to slow the bowels down as they are just now gearing up. So, I spent most of Thursday night in the bathroom. Thankfully,

I left a magazine in there earlier in the day as I had plenty of time to read in the middle of the night.

Friday evening. 72 hours post-op. I actually had a diarrhea-free day. However, my stomach is very swollen, assuming the appearance of a basketball. The incisions look good; and my newly recharged colon has gone into overdrive in the gas-production department! I think I'll stay at home for a while.

I truly believe the reason my colon went right to work and I was able to come home so quickly, and the reason I have had surprisingly little pain following this surgery, is a direct result of prayer.

Saturday April 10, 2010

Diarrhea + Silk duvet cover = Poor combination

Recent abdominal surgery + Sprinting to the bathroom = Poor combination

Laughter + God's mercy = Perfect combination!

Friday night was much the same as Thursday night, lots of time in the bathroom. It makes me think of an infant who has nights and days mixed up. Not exactly, but my system certainly has night and day confused.

Saturday morning was calm, only to be followed by Saturday afternoon's frenzied sprints to the bathroom. This is not much fun, but I guess I am making progress. Maybe this afternoon's fun means I will actually get to sleep tonight.

I am a little worried about the carpet between my bed and the bathroom; maybe I should pull it up until things have settled down.

Whose idea was this? Thankfully I am still able to laugh.

Gotta run!

Sunday April 11, 2010
Rest Once More

I was reading my Bible Tuesday morning before going to the hospital and God spoke to me these words: *"Let my soul be at rest again, for the Lord has been good to me." Psalm 116:7 (NLT)*

Such sweet words to encourage me as I went to have my final surgery.

I have been trying to hold on to those words through this recovery. This recovery has been hard for me physically and emotionally. I've had very little pain at the surgical site, but the loss of bowel control has taken its toll. It's just not a problem you ever want to experience - the words "embarrassing" and "humiliating" come to mind.

Saturday evening was full of tears. I am still coming to grips with the idea that things will never be exactly the same again. I will always be a cancer survivor. I will always experience the long-term side effects of radiation and surgery. I've been told that, and I know it intellectually, but I am just beginning to process it emotionally.

Today, with every step I feel the irritated nerves in my feet. Only God knows how long that will last. With every use of my hands I am made aware of the numbness of my fingertips. Will it ever go away? Every look in the mirror I see a stooped, tired little girl.

Then God steps in.

- I read these words in *Jesus Calling*: "Trust me in every detail of your life... Having sacrificed my very life for you, I can be trusted in every facet of your life."
- I remember that I actually slept through the night. Saturday night. That is definitely progress.

- I receive a note from a sweet friend reminding me that I am a warrior.
- I have the joy of watching Community of Faith's worship service live on the Internet.
- I find a website with encouraging information about recovery from ileostomy reversal surgery. It seems my bowels are right on track! I actually feel somewhat more in control today.
- Phone calls, messages, and texts from friends and family come throughout the day reminding me of their love and prayers.
- Mark and I walk 1.3 miles around the lake behind our house. It took me a while, but I made it. It was so nice to enjoy the sunset, the flowers, the breeze, the ducks, and time with my husband!
- Dinner brought by sweet friends, Erica, Brooke, and Brea. Those beautiful faces would make anyone feel better!

The Lord has indeed been good to me! He gave me this day full of His blessings! I will rest once more.

Monday April 12, 2010
Simple Pleasures

I am making progress. Today has been a good day. No sprints to the bathroom, so far, at least.

Mark and I spent the morning hanging out together, which is always fun. I actually spent a little while out in the sun today. I walked out of the bedroom in an old swim suit, one that I knew would cover my stomach without any seams or anything that would put pressure on my incision, and asked Mark, while posing, "Well, what do you think?" He took one look at my new bird-legs, basketball-belly, and pasty-skinned form and started to laugh. I love his honesty. I started to laugh, too, as I held on to my sore belly. Laughter feels good. No telling what the neighbors thought of me out by the pool.

The doorbell rang later and we opened the door to the delivery of an edible bouquet from some sweet friends. The bouquet had (notice the use of past tense here) chocolate covered strawberries in it as well as purple grapes - my favorite! And then it hit me, I can eat grapes again! I don't have to avoid the skins anymore. The ileostomy is gone. Mark and I enjoyed a great afternoon snack.

Simple pleasures are always the best.

"But I am trusting you, O Lord. saying, 'You are my God!'" Psalm 31:14 (NLT)

Wednesday April 14, 2010
Bathroom Marathon

Tuesday, not so good. My bowel system is going from one extreme to the other, which is apparently a normal development following the type of surgery I've had. It also goes from relatively normal days to days of sheer panic to get to the bathroom. Also a very typical response for this type of surgery. It makes it a little hard to plan anything or go anywhere because I never know when or how the nightmare will begin.

And by nightmare, I mean nightmare. Tuesday was going relatively well - one round of bathroom marathon in the afternoon. Then around 6:00 Tuesday evening it started all over again. I spent three hours in and out of the bathroom every 5-10 minutes. Literally. Three hours. I never understood the reason for a bidet in the bathroom, but now I do. I so wished I had one last night. A garden hose would have been acceptable at that point.

My plan is to strangle the surgeon when I go see him on Friday. I know it's not his fault, but it feels good to have someone to blame!

By 8:00 p.m. I am in tears thinking about the fact that I can't take any medication to stop this, and I think to myself, "My bowels will be the death of me." That thought struck me to the core, realizing the fact that my bowels may very well be the cause of my death one day. I crumble to the bathroom floor in a heap, sobbing in anger, fear, and grief.

Then I remember that I am a warrior. I struggle back to my feet shouting, "No! No! No! No!" I will not let my enemy get the best of me tonight. Then God softly whispers, "I am here. You can do this. There is no death for you, only life. I've already paid the price. I have given you life. You have life."

He's always here when I need Him. He never leaves. He even hangs out in my bathroom!

"... but even in darkness I cannot hide from you. To you the night shines as bright as day. Darkness and light are the same to you." Psalm 139:12 (NLT)

Wednesday April 14, 2010
Top 10 Rules to Live By When You Have a Short Rectum

God is always faithful to encourage me through my friends. He has used many to be the hands and feet and hugs of Jesus to me. Just yesterday a sweet friend delivered fresh corn bread to my front door. Today, another friend surprised me with a giant package of Charmin toilet paper! And then I received the following advice from a new friend who has walked this path before me.

Top 10 Rules to Live By When You Have a Short Rectum

1. Always wear underwear.

2. Know where the nearest bathroom is at all times. In Times Square, it is at McDonald's.

3. Keep lots of reading materials and a digital Yahtzee game in the bathroom.

4. If you don't have reading materials readily available, don't stop on the way to the bathroom to get them. You will not have time.

5. A hot shower does wonders for your state of mind.

6. When needed, a heated chamomile-scented rice bag on your rump is very relaxing and takes the edge off.

7. Spending time in your bathroom with God is sometimes the only place He can get you still. Just talk to Him and discover what a blessing it is.

8. Don't wear white pants unless you are having a really good day and you haven't eaten anything.

9. Make some phone calls from the bathroom. No one has to know that your colon is under construction, especially the PET scan receptionist or the insurance representative.

10. Last but not least, God is in control, even when you are not, literally!

Thanks to my friends, today has been a much better day.

Monday April 19, 2010
New Routines

I had an appointment with the surgeon last Friday. He removed my stitches. I shared with him my bathroom adventures from the previous ten days. He says that everything is on schedule and that it will take two to three months for things to establish a new normal routine. The nerves in the section of my colon that were reattached are learning their new job, and that takes a little bit of time.

Having said all that, I am happy to report that it seems for now things have already settled into a new normal routine. I know there may be some more non-routine days in the weeks ahead, but I think for the most part my intestines have adjusted quite well.

I am able to eat a regular high-fiber diet now. I can drive and swim. I don't have to go back to see the surgeon for another month.

Tuesday April 20, 2010
Signs of Life

I've been thinking about scars lately. We all have them, in some form or fashion. Some are physical, some are emotional, but all of us carry them with us. And it's our choice what we will do with them. We can choose to let them constantly remind us of the pain we've experienced, to hold us captive to the past; or we can choose to let them remind us of our victories and take strength and courage from them to move forward.

In the past eleven months I have gained five new scars on my body. I was actually opened up in six different places, but one of them went through an old abdominal scar, so only five new scars. If you connect the dots on my belly, it actually forms a smile, with one large dimple!

Scars, for me, are signs of life. I've been in the battle, I fought for my life, I fought for my family, and I won! Bring on the scars! They just remind me that God has been good to me. His mercy, kindness, and never-ending grace left me with scars – signs of life, and I am grateful.

Newsflash: I zipped *and* buttoned my jeans for the first time in eight months today!

Friday April 23, 2010
Remain in Him

For some reason it is taking me a while to actually get my brain back into gear and get on with my life. I'm sure this is a normal response after all the stress we've been through the past year, but it feels weird. Now that I am free of constant medical appointments, free of constant fatigue, free of medications and inconvenient side effects, I still feel like I am stuck here. I can't quite seem to get my "To Do" list made, which has never been a problem in my life before.

I was thinking about this last week and asking God for help in this area. After He stopped laughing at my idea of making a "To Do" list, He spoke to my heart. He told me that I had been looking at things all wrong. I am not Laura Shook, girl who had cancer. I am Laura Shook, disciple of God. God has used cancer to teach me and train me and make me more like Jesus, but it doesn't define who I am. I am still a disciple of God.

Nothing has changed really. I'm still me. All I have to do is keep walking with God; keep looking to Him to direct me and guide me.

Just today these thoughts were reinforced as I read the following Scriptures:

"But my eyes are fixed on you, O Sovereign Lord; in you I take refuge – do not give me over to death." Psalm 141:8 (NIV)

"Live in me. Make your home in me just as I do in you. In the same way that a branch can't bear grapes by itself but only by being joined to the vine, you can't bear fruit unless you are joined with me. I am the Vine, you are the branches. When you're joined with me and I with you,

the relation is intimate and organic, the harvest is sure to be abundant. Separated, you can't produce a thing." John 15:4-5 (The Message)

Spending time with God, remaining in Him, fixing my eyes on Him, is the single most important thing I can do today. It is the greatest need that I have; and if I will put that at the top of the list, everything else will fall into place.

Thanks for reminding me, Lord, that this is about so much more than a girl who had cancer. It's about You and Your Kingdom. Please help me to remain in You.

Tuesday April 27, 2010
Ordinary Life

I love to watch the sunrise. I love the stillness and quiet of the morning, the anticipation of a new day and all the promise that it holds. In the early morning calm I am reminded that God is here and that He cares. The sunrise brings with it the chance for a fresh start, a new beginning, and renewed strength for whatever the day brings. I am grateful that God knew we would need these new starts, and that we would need them frequently.

Now that there are no kids in the house I don't see the sunrise very often. Mark and I don't have to get up before dawn to make breakfast or pack lunches or drive kids to school. And we miss those moments - the miraculous turning of the sky from black to brilliant hues of pink and orange - those moments that confirm that God is indeed a God of goodness and mercy, a God of new beginnings!

I haven't seen the sunrise lately, but I have seen the dawn of a new day in my life. For the first time in nearly a year, I have felt relatively normal. I feel good physically. I am not tired. I can eat. I can leave the house. I have been successful at rejecting fearful and worrisome thoughts. I feel the sun rising!

Mark and I are enjoying ordinary life. Friday night we attended the Astros game with my parents. The Astros won, and we stayed all the way through the fireworks at the end of the game.

Saturday I actually worked in the yard! I can't remember the last time I had my hands in the dirt. It felt good to be in the sun, using muscles I haven't used in a long time. I'm not sure my surgeon would have been too happy, but he wasn't here.

Sunday night I went swimming. I haven't been in a pool in a year!

I read this quote from Katherine Rich, a cancer survivor, in the *New York Times* today: "All I wanted was ordinary life back, for ordinary life, it became utterly clear, is more valuable than anything else."

Thank You, Lord, for giving me my ordinary life back. Please help me never to take that blessing for granted.

Maybe I'll get up and watch the sunrise tomorrow.

Wednesday April 28, 2010
Enjoy the Ride

This week I've been thinking about the fact that God wants to be in control of our lives; and the idea that we have to recognize and allow Him to be in control.

I started picturing what it would be like if I was riding in the car as a passenger and didn't realize that Mark was actually driving. What would happen? Well, as soon as I thought that no one was in control of the car I would have jumped into the driver's seat and shoved Mark out of the way, preventing him from driving. I would have grabbed the steering wheel, jerking the car out of its lane and into oncoming traffic. As the car veered out of control I would have suddenly pulled the emergency brake, sending the car into a totally uncontrolled spin all while still trying to kick Mark out of the way. I would have been dodging other cars on the road, trying to avoid mowing down pedestrians. Finally, screaming after a long struggle, my emotions off the scale, sweat dripping down my forehead and tears in my eyes I would have finally brought the car to a complete standstill facing the wrong direction. Then I would have looked at Mark and screamed, "Why didn't you control the car?"

Of course, that's not ever really going to happen. If I am a passenger in the car I can plainly see who is in control. I know who's driving. I'm not tempted to jump into the driver's seat and take over. Doing so would only lead to disaster. But how many times do I do just that in my life? I fail to remember that God is in control, or maybe I don't want Him in control, thinking I can do things better; and I jump in, push Him out of the way, grab the wheel and begin the struggle to control a careening life. How much wiser would it be to look to Him, see that He is God, He is good, He is in control? Then I can just sit back and enjoy the ride!

"You alone are the God who is in heaven. You are ruler of all the kingdoms of the earth. You are powerful and mighty; no one an stand against you!" 2 Chronicles 20:6 (NLT)

That's who I want in control in my life, the One that no one can defeat!

Thursday April 29, 2010
Long-term

Tomorrow is my birthday. Yes, 29 again. My driver's license expires on my birthday this year, which is OK since I happen to have lost it. I know it's in this house somewhere.

So today I went to renew my license. I wasn't too excited about going and having my picture taken. I look OK in person, but with my hair so thin now (Yes, it's still falling out!) I just don't look good in pictures. This is the license I will have to carry with me for the next ten years.

I drove out to the Department of Public Safety office. There were only two people ahead of me in line, and the ladies who work in this office were friendly and efficient. They gave me a vision test. Thankfully I passed. They asked me how much I weigh - a lot less than last time! They scanned my thumbprints; and then they told me to step back against the wall to take my picture. I was feeling OK until she handed me my receipt and my temporary license, which actually had the picture on it. So, yeah, I still look like a cancer patient. Or maybe a scarecrow?

But here's the good news. I actually thought long-term today! I was thinking of having and using this license for ten years. I have moved past the five-year time frame! And the other good news is I realized I only have to keep this license for six years, not ten like I originally thought.

Monday May 3, 2010

I have been feeling really well lately in every way. But every few days, at the most unexpected times, I have a mini-meltdown. Unusual things will bring up grief and a longing for how things used to be. For all these months I have been hoping to "get my life back" and now I am discovering that that's not going to happen exactly. Yes, I will get my usual routines back, but they won't be the same anymore. Everything has changed. At times it feels like I am falling without a net, not sure where I will end up, and not sure how to stop the fall. Little things occasionally still overwhelm me. And so goes recovery from cancer. Moment-by-moment, day-by-day, seeking and trusting God to provide answers, direction, encouragement, and comfort.

I am reminded that life is a series of changes. When nothing is changing, there is nothing living. I like that thought. Change equals life. So I will embrace change and choose to live.

Thursday May 6, 2010
Stand Firm

One of my favorite stories in the Bible is a story found in 2 Chronicles about King Jehoshaphat. I have always loved this story because it is a story of God's power at work in the life of His people. Several armies had banded together and were coming against King Jehoshaphat. Instead of running in fear, or surrendering to the enemy, listen to what Jehoshaphat chose to do:

"We will stand in your presence…and will cry out to you in our distress, and you will hear us and save us…For we have no power to face this vast army that is attacking us. We do not know what to do, but our eyes are upon you.

And they stood there before the Lord." 2 Chronicles 20:9,12,13 (NIV)

When I was first diagnosed with cancer it took my breath away. I didn't know what to do, how to react, how to respond, how to move. And I remember praying that same prayer one day: I don't know what to do, but my eyes are on You.

"I will stand in Your presence" became my battle cry. No matter what happens, I will stand and declare that You are God. I might not be able to do anything else, but I'll stand and declare that I am Yours, come what may.

When Jehoshaphat and the people of Israel stood before the Lord listen to what God said to them:

"Do not be afraid or discouraged because of this vast army. For the battle is not yours, but God's… Take up your positions; stand firm and see the deliverance the Lord will give you… Then

Jehoshaphat bowed with his face to the ground and all the people
of Judah and Jerusalem fell down in worship before the Lord."
2 Chronicles 20:15,17,18 *(NIV)*

I love that! God's people focused their eyes on Him and they
stood. They stood there and watched God perform a miracle.
They stood there and watched God win the victory. And then they
bowed to the ground to worship this great God!

A beautiful story of an even more beautiful God. I choose to
worship Him today. He is a God of victory!

Sunday May 9, 2010
Relay for Life

Friday afternoon Mark and I hopped in the car and headed out to
the nearby town of Waller, Texas, for the Waller County Relay for
Life. Every year the whole town comes together to raise money
for the American Cancer Society to fund research to find cures for
cancer.

This was the first time I had ever participated in such
an event. I was given a purple t-shirt to wear with the word
SURVIVOR in large white letters on the back. As soon as I arrived
at the stadium people greeted me and congratulated me. It felt
like we were family. I registered at the Survivors table and was
given a bag full of gifts.

The Boy Scouts presented the colors, a local high school
student sang the national anthem, and Mark opened the event
with prayer. All the survivors lined up at the fifty-yard line to
be recognized. I won the prize for "Most Recently Diagnosed"
and was given a sash to wear, as if I were Miss America! And
then, with the song "I'm a Survivor" blaring over the speakers,
we made our way around the track. It was a surreal moment. I
was walking with the cancer survivors. It was hard to believe,

especially since I still have a hard time believing I actually had cancer. People were standing around the track with balloons, cheering for us as we walked by. Luminaries lined the track in memory of those who have gone before us, and in honor of those who fought the battle and won.

So many thoughts and emotions filled my heart and my head, but mostly I felt incredibly grateful. So grateful for God's faithfulness and His goodness. So grateful for amazing friends who have loved and supported me. So grateful for my family. So grateful to be alive.

Thursday May 13, 2010
The Rear View

Mark and I have lived in nineteen different homes in the years that we've been married. In spite of that awesome number of moves, I have never driven a moving truck. Until yesterday, that is. I helped our daughter move to a new city to start her first full-time job after college graduation.

One of the most interesting things about driving a moving truck is that you can't see out the back of the truck. In fact, there isn't even a rearview mirror in the truck, because there is no view. While I was driving the truck I discovered that I have a well-established habit of using my rearview mirror when I drive. I can't tell you how many times I tried to check the rearview mirror only to find that there was no mirror and no view.

While I was driving and checking the non-existent mirror God whispered to my heart, "Don't look back." He caught me by surprise but I knew it was His voice. I still struggle at times focusing on cancer instead of living my life, wondering what I could have done to prevent this, or what I can do now to ensure long-term survival. All these thoughts bring anxiety and I have been asking God to help me let it all go, to choose to continue to trust Him, and to move on. The same way it was useless for me to try to look back while driving the truck, it is useless for me to look back at this point in my life. God wants me to look forward; and so He used my truck driving experience to bring it home to my heart. Don't look back.

Monday May 17, 2010
For the Record

I had a post-surgery follow-up visit with the surgeon today. After filling my bowels with air and inserting various fun exam instruments, he told me that everything has healed well and looks good. Each time I hear a positive report my heart feels a little lighter. I don't have to see the surgeon again for three months, when we will schedule my next colonoscopy – always something fun with him!

Just for the record, as the doctor was examining my surgical site, he asked me to raise my head so that he could feel the muscle strength around the former ileostomy site. Then he said, and I quote, "Your muscles are strong." I started laughing, thinking he must be kidding. He assured me that he was serious. I have good abdominal strength. So, I just want everyone to know that it has been confirmed by a top notch, highly degreed medical professional that I have six-pack abs! OK, maybe that's not exactly what he said, but he might as well have said it that way because that's how I'm taking it!

I hopped in the car to drive home from the doctor's office and the lyrics "Glory, honor, and power belong to You" were playing on the radio. It seemed so appropriate today and I sang praises and smiled all the way home.

Tuesday May 18, 2010
Lesson Learned

Don't go to a group fitness class on the same day that you have air pumped into your intestines. Your friends will thank you.

Wednesday May 19, 2010
Passport to Intimacy

I recently heard a quote by Bruce Feiler, the author of *The Council of Dads*. Mr. Feiler was diagnosed with bone cancer in 2008 at the age of 43. At the time, his twin daughters were three years old. As he contemplated the uncertainty of his future, Mr. Feiler created the "Council of Dads" to provide stability and support that his girls may need over the years. Thankfully, Mr. Feiler is alive and well today, and the relationships that have developed between him, his wife, his daughters, and this special group of friend dads has enriched all of their lives. Mr. Feiler said, "Cancer is a passport to intimacy." I smiled when I heard this because it confirmed my thoughts exactly.

One of the side effects of cancer has been a deepening of relationships all around - with Mark, with my kids, with my parents, my brothers, and my friends. Learning (or being forced) to admit your weaknesses and fears goes a long way in forming strong bonds between two people. Asking for and accepting help from others establishes a sweet knowing and connection between two people. A diagnosis of cancer strips away all the shallow and superficial ways we relate to one another and provides the perfect canvas on which to build a foundation of intimacy. It causes you to see clearly what really matters in this life. I have loved and been loved like I never have before. I'm so glad God chose me to walk this path with Him!

"He is intimate with the upright." Proverbs 3:32 (NASB)

Saturday May 22, 2010
The Blue Dress

I was ironing a dress today (Yes, you read that right. It doesn't happen often, but occasionally I do iron.) when I remembered that it was the dress I often wore to go to the radiation center. I wore it because it was easy to change in and out of, making those appointments a little less complicated. I slowly ironed, remembering those early days of treatment – the shock, the uncertainty and fear, the anger, the grief, and finally the peace that came as I chose to trust my Savior's heart.

So much has happened over these months, and it all happened so quickly that it's hard to remember it all. And I desperately want to remember. I want to remember everything that happened, every thought, every feeling. And more than anything I want to remember all God taught me. I want to be able to use these things to help someone else. So, that's my prayer.

Lord, please keep this experience fresh in my mind. Please take this experience and use it for Your Kingdom and Your Glory. I am available to You.

Monday May 24, 2010
Strange and Wonderful

I have started referring to the past year as the missing year. It feels like my normal life paused on May 27, 2009, and wasn't resumed until just recently. The year of cancer was just stuck in there. I notice the missing year often now, especially when I am out in the community or talking to people I haven't seen in a while. There are new businesses I haven't seen, restaurants I haven't visited, information and activities that I missed. I feel pretty normal until one of these situations comes up, and then I am reminded that I had cancer, I missed a year.

On one of the pages in my 2009 journal there is an unusual list. This list is called "Things I have missed." The list includes specific parties and events, worship services, meetings, trips, foods, funerals, celebrations, and activities with friends. It seems funny now, that I was keeping a list of everything I missed. But it is a stark reminder of the way that cancer invades and takes over every area of your life, not just your physical life. Cancer is uninvited, unwelcome, and it eats away at everything. It changes everything.

As difficult as that experience was, it also forms the backdrop that allows me to enjoy each new day and every new experience now. Every time I am able to visit with a friend, attend a party, go to church, or hang out with my family, I am so grateful for the opportunity to do so.

I went to the gym today for the first time in a year. It felt strange and wonderful to actually be out in the world doing things that normal people do instead of sitting in hospital and doctor waiting rooms.

Strange because it feels like I've been gone for a long time and the world went on without me. Strange because I don't have an answer for people who don't know where I've been this past year and innocently say to me, "I haven't seen you here in a while."

But wonderful because I feel like I am finally emerging from a fog. Wonderful because I am alive. Wonderful because I am healthy!

As I sit on the weight bench testing my long dormant muscles, I marvel at the fact that I am there and I am healthy. I watch all the people exercising and wonder if any of them have cancer. I hope they are aware of the blessing of their health.

I'm sure I will be sore tomorrow; but as I crawl out of bed in the morning and feel the ache of my muscles, I will praise God for every twinge, for He has been good to me and I know it!

"Open your mouth and taste, open your eyes and see – how good God is. Blessed are you who run to him." Psalm 34:8

Tuesday May 25, 2010
The Broken Watch

My watch died about the same time I was diagnosed with cancer last year. Ordinarily I am one of those people who live by a calendar and a schedule. A broken watch should have thrown my world into chaos, but it seems that had already been accomplished by the three little words, "You have cancer." Due to all the turmoil that ensued, I never replaced my watch. I have lived without one for over a year now, and I kind of like it.

I find that I am less stressed. I move more slowly. I don't rush to accomplish things. I take time to enjoy people and conversations and nature and quiet. I was thinking about this strange new way of life for me today and wondered if maybe this is in some small way how Jesus lived his life on this earth. I don't imagine He was ever stressed. He knew that everything was ultimately in God's loving hands. I don't think He rushed from town to town. He took His time, stopping to talk to people, to hug children, to heal the sick, to teach the crowds. I don't think He was worried about accomplishing anything except what God gave Him to do that day – no one to please, no one to impress – His whole goal to fulfill God's plan for the day.

I've been thinking about buying a new watch, but the more I think about it, maybe I won't.

"So I commend the enjoyment of life, because there is nothing better for people under the sun than to eat and drink and be glad. Then joy will accompany them in their toil all the days of the life God has given them under the sun." Ecclesiastes 8:15 (NIV)

Wednesday June 16, 2010
Just Thinking

I was just thinking today. During the whole time that I was sick and focused on fighting a deadly enemy, life went on without me. Mark continued to go to work, the kids went to school, Community of Faith continued on. The only thing that mattered during that time was my relationship with Christ. I was desperate to have Him close, to know He was with me, to hear His words, and to be comforted and strengthened by his presence. He gave me life and hope. He was all I needed. It was the only thing that mattered.

Now that life is going on *with* me, shouldn't it still be the same? My relationship with Christ should still be the one thing that really matters. If I keep that my focus then everything else will fall into place.

"It is not circumstances that need altering first, but yourselves, and then the conditions will naturally alter. Spare no effort to become all I would have you. Follow every leading. I am your only Guide."
(*God Calling*)

Sunday June 20, 2010
Island of Misfits

Remember *Rudolph the Red-Nosed Reindeer and the Island of Misfit Toys*? Lately I have been feeling like a misfit. In *Rudolph*, this island is where all the defective and unwanted toys are sent. While I don't think I am defective or unwanted, I sure do feel like a misfit. I feel like a very different person than the one who began this whole cancer journey. And I still struggle to find my place in my own life now!

I keep thinking I should just be happy that I am healthy and get to keep living; and most days I feel great. But then there are moments like these when the tears come again, or the anger, or the grief.

I had such a good week and so many good things happened, and I saw God's hand at work. And then today I feel like a misfit. I'm just different. I feel most at home when I am with other cancer survivors. There is an immediate kinship between us, a knowing.

I am one of the dwindling few who still read the Sunday newspaper. I was feeling these things again today when I opened up the *Houston Chronicle* and found *Parade Magazine*, which had a special report called "Cancer in America." According to the article, I'm not the only cancer survivor who feels like a misfit. Maybe we all do.

"But let all who take refuge in you be glad; let them ever sing for joy. Spread your protection over them, that those who love your name may rejoice in you. For surely, O Lord, you bless the righteous, you surround them with your favor as with a shield." Psalm 5:11-12 (NIV)

Monday June 21, 2010
All Systems Go!

I had an appointment with the oncologist today. It had been three months since my last visit. As I drove to his office today I realized that I wasn't nervous or worried at all. I fully expected all the reports to be good today.

It was strange to walk into the building. It brought back so many memories, not all pleasant, and it was great to walk in feeling good! I saw some of my "chemo friends" today - still coming to the office for regular chemotherapy treatments, still experiencing uncomfortable side effects, still fighting for one more day of life. How thankful I am that those days are behind me! I am reminded to pray for these sweet friends daily.

The doctor reviewed all my lab work and test results, performed a physical exam, and then declared that everything is normal. I'm normal. He said that he would order another PET scan for September to make sure that I am still disease-free.

As I left his office and started the drive home I began to think about the PET scan planned for September, and the fact that we won't know if there has been any recurrence until that time. Suddenly, the fear monster reared his head and threatened to take over. I started doing deep breathing exercises, telling myself the truth. As I did so, I heard God whisper to my heart, "I got this." Immediately the fear disappeared and a huge smile spread across my face. My God has this under control. The almighty, all-knowing, all-loving, faithful creator of all things has me in His hands.

I felt like shouting all the way home. I'm pretty sure my feet never touched the ground for the rest of the day!

Wednesday August 11, 2010
Physically, Emotionally, Spiritually

It has now been four months since my last surgery. Physically, I feel great. I feel strong. All is settled with my bowel system. I am able to eat a normal diet with just a few off-limits foods (nuts, popcorn, and chips) that seem to mess me up when I eat them. The numbness caused by irritated nerves in my fingertips and feet continues to incrementally improve.

Emotionally, I am on the mend. I have had several weird emotional days with lots of tears. I think I am finally able to release some of the things that were suppressed while I was busy fighting this disease, so that has been a positive experience. I had a few days during the past month when the reality that I am healthy and alive crashed through and brought me to my knees in gratitude. Again, another positive experience! There are still moments when I experience some survivor's guilt, and moments when fear tries to creep in. I have become adept at recognizing those moments and those thoughts and choosing instead to continue to trust that everything is in God's hands.

Spiritually, I am a different person than I was fifteen months ago. I have a deep peace. I don't worry anymore, or at least not for long. I was reading in 2 Timothy the other day and came across a verse that I have known forever, but for some reason, this time I read it differently: *"...I know the one in whom I trust, and I am sure that he is able to guard what I have entrusted to him until the day of his return."* 2 Timothy 1:12 (NLT)

I have always read this verse as "I know who it is I am trusting," as in I know His name, I know who He is. But when I read it this time, it was different. I don't just know who He is; I don't just know His name, I know *Him.* I am intimately connected with my Savior. In the past year, through the darkest of times, I learned things about God's character that I can't even begin to express in words. I committed my life to Him years ago, but in the past year I saw in a very real way how He is committed to me. That is incomprehensible to me. Now He is absolutely everything to me. "I *know* the one in whom I trust..."

I read these words recently: "... no man can see my face and live. The self, the original man, shrivels up and dies, and upon the soul becomes stamped my image." (*God Calling*)

I feel like that's what cancer has done. It has allowed me a tiny glimpse of the face of God – His sovereignty, His kindness, His power, His love, and His mercy. And maybe that's the change I sense in me, and have heard mentioned by so many other cancer patients and survivors. "I'm different now." " Everything has changed." Maybe it's that glimpse of God and His image now stamped on our souls.

Tuesday August 17, 2010
Surveillance

I had an appointment with the surgeon yesterday. He talked about the fact that we are in surveillance mode now. We discussed how important it is to have regular surveillance in order to make sure I am healthy. He reminded me that if rectal cancer recurs, it most often occurs within the first two years after the initial diagnosis; and it most often returns at the site of the original tumor, or in the liver or the lungs. I didn't really want to be reminded of those things. I don't like to focus on that possibility, but I guess it is good to remember. So, we have a four-part surveillance plan in place:

1. Vigilance - I have to pay attention to my body and listen to it. If I experience any of the symptoms of colorectal cancer – bleeding, excessive gas, change in bowel habits, abdominal pain – I need to report those symptoms to my doctor right away.
2. Physical Exam - I will see my surgeon and my oncologist every three months to be examined. Exams include blood work, and all the instruments of torture that I have discussed before.
3. Colonoscopy - I will have an annual colonoscopy for several years.
4. Scans - My surgeon agrees that the best scan for me is the PET scan. Unless something changes, a scan will be ordered every six months.

When I saw the doctor yesterday, this is how our conversation went:

Doctor: "How are you feeling?"

Me: "I feel good!"

Doctor: "Are you feeling strong?"

Me: "Yes, I feel strong!" I reply, thinking that's a good way to describe it.

Doctor: "You *look* strong,"

And I wonder, is "strong" doctor-speak for "You've gained weight"?

Thursday August 19, 2010
Spoke Too Soon

At the surgeon's office on Monday he asks me, "Do you have complete control of your bowels now?" It has been four months since surgery to close the ileostomy.

"Yes!" I proudly respond.

On Wednesday afternoon, I am shopping with Sarah when I suddenly realize that I spoke too soon. I run to the restroom and to my horror discover that bowel control may still be an occasional issue. Thankfully we are in a department store. I stroll over to the women's clothes, choose a package of underwear and casually change clothes in the restroom. I'm not sure what the sales lady thought as I purchased an open package of underwear, but Sarah and I certainly made a crazy memory today!

Monday August 23, 2010
Divine Love

Last week I was reading my Bible and came across an incredible verse. I'd read it before, but for some reason it really hit me this time. Maybe it was the translation I was using, or maybe it was just something God wanted me to see now.

"*Yet I still dare to hope when I remember this: the faithful love of the Lord never ends! His mercies never cease."* Lamentations 3:21-22 (NLT)

I love that! His love *never* ends! His mercies *never* stop!

Have you ever turned on the faucet in your bathtub, and then got busy and walked away and forgot to turn it off? That's what this verse makes me think of. It's as if I have a cup and a bottomless pitcher. I start to pour into the cup, I keep pouring and I never stop. Imagine that. First the water would fill up the cup, it would get to the brim, and then it would spill over. It would begin to run out over the table, and then spill over the edge, getting the carpet wet until it was saturated. It would trickle across the floor and begin to fill up the room, eventually making its way out the door and down to the street.

That's how God's love is. That's how His mercy is. It *never* ends. God *never* turns it off. It is constantly pouring out all over me, filling me up; and then it spills out of me onto everything and everyone around me. It's like a faucet that is never turned off.

And water, poured out, changes things. It moves things, It covers things. It carves rivers and canyons. God's love, continually poured out, does the same thing. It changes us, it moves us, it covers a multitude of sins, it carves the landscape of our lives so that things are never the same. That has been my experience with cancer.

What an amazing gift - divine love poured onto me, continually, daily, surrounding me, covering me, carrying me, changing me! Thank You, Lord, for Your mercies that never stop. Let it pour!

Monday September 6, 2010
Anticipation

I have been drinking clear liquids today, getting ready for tomorrow's colonoscopy. The day brings with it lots of memories.

Memories of that first colonoscopy in May 2009. Memories of the shock and chaos that ensued. I pull out the pictures of the tumor and still find it hard to believe it was living inside of me and I was unaware.

This colonoscopy will be the first one I've had since I was diagnosed with cancer. I am anxious to hear the doctor's report. Looking forward to hearing that the surgery site looks great; there are no polyps, no tumors, no inflamed lymph nodes; and that my colon is completely healthy.

I'm off to start drinking HalfLytely and making runs to the bathroom. Yuck! I've already tried to convince Mark that this is the last colonoscopy I will ever need, but he isn't going for it.

Tuesday September 7, 2010
Normal Colon

Today's colonoscopy went well. Afterward, the doctor came in smiling. He said everything looked good. My colon was clear - no polyps, no cancer, and the surgical site looks great. He gave us pictures of my colon, which look markedly different from last year's pictures. The surgical staples are even visible.

Then I read these words at the end of the report: "Normal Colon."

I can't even tell you the joy that flooded my heart! I have a normal colon. God has been good to me!

Sunday September 12, 2010
Spring Cleaning in the Fall

After I was diagnosed with cancer, Mark and I seemed to miss summer, fall, winter, and spring. Cancer treatment was at the top of the priority list, and there was nothing else on the list. All the usual things fell by the wayside. Home maintenance, yard maintenance, cleaning, laundry, and repairs - anything that wasn't directly related to cancer treatment just didn't happen.

Now that treatment is behind us, it feels like we are beginning to emerge from a cocoon. Slowly, I am digging out from under the piles of paperwork that have been left to build over the past year. I have begun the unpleasant project of cleaning out the garage. You can imagine how fun that is after fifteen months of not being swept or cleaned at all - lots of little critters are living there. I am getting rid of old clothes and unused household items; cleaning out drawers and cabinets. I even decided to clean the windows. I woke up Sunday morning, sore all over, and loving it!

The amazing thing is how good it feels. I actually have the strength and stamina to do these things! I can carry boxes. I can climb ladders. I can push and pull and sweep and scrub. And I am so happy to do so. Cancer definitely changes your perspective on things!

Every mundane task has new significance now. The ordinary chores of daily living bring joy. I feel like I am seeing things for the first time again, as if through the eyes of a child, full of wonder at the beauty of life. I am alive! Thank you, God, for new eyes to see the beauty of life.

One of the songs we sang at church today has the line, "I can't bow low enough..." And that's exactly how I feel now. I can't bow low enough. I can't begin to express my gratitude to God for what He's done in my life. For now, I'll just keep singing, and cleaning, smiling, and enjoying every new day.

"I can't bow low enough
I can't bow low enough
at the vision of You my God
I can't hold it all inside
I'm reaching for the One who brought me out of death and

into life
but I can't lift my hands high enough
lift my hands high enough
when I'm reaching for You my God
I can't lift my hands high enough
lift my hands high enough
when I'm reaching for You my God
oh I'm reaching for You my God"
("Cielo," by Phil Wickham)

Tuesday September 14, 2010
Not Finished Yet

Since finishing treatment and surgery, it has been interesting to me how many people have expressed their pleasure that I am all finished with cancer and I don't have to deal with it anymore.

I just smile and acknowledge their kind hearts, but the truth is I'm not finished yet. Not even close. Yes, I am finished with the immediate treatment. Yes, I am finished with surgery. But I'm not finished with cancer. In fact, it seems like just recently the stress of the past fifteen months is beginning to surface in me, Mark, and our girls. My husband and my children have all been so strong, pushing their own feelings aside in order to carry me through treatment. Now that it looks like I am well, the defenses are dropping and the feelings are surfacing. We are all feeling a little fragile at this point.

I think about cancer every day. I have physical changes and new routines that remind me of where I've been on a daily basis. Although they are less frequent now, I still have regular doctor visits and medical tests. I still take multiple dietary supplements prescribed by my doctor to treat side effects of chemotherapy. Cancer is still part of my daily life.

I had a PET scan today. I didn't feel nervous at all about the test or the results of the test. Mark took me to the radiology center and patiently waited two hours. Afterward we stopped to pick up lunch on the way to our staff meeting. Returning to the car I suddenly felt extremely fatigued. I realized that although I hadn't felt it, I must have been stressed all along. Mark got in the car and told me that he was having a mini-meltdown too. Even though we fully believe that I am cancer-free, the waiting, hoping, and wondering are heavy loads to carry. Hopefully, the doctor will call soon with the report.

In the meantime, we'll carry on, as survivors. Never forgetting where we've been, and ever look forward to God's continued grace and strength.

Thursday September 16, 2010
Hair Update

Our dog Biscuit is a Maltese. If he were well groomed, he would have a long, soft, shiny white coat of hair. This beautiful topcoat would cover the undercoat of shorter hair that grows close to his skin.

One of our cats, Shadow, has a long, thick coat of shiny black hair. Most of the year it looks like velvet until she starts shedding in the summer. If she is not brushed daily her gorgeous coat becomes a mess with the hair matting with her undercoat.

I never really gave much thought to the fact that my precious pets had a topcoat of fur and an undercoat of fur. That is until I noticed the same thing happening on my head. I was so happy when my hair stopped falling out. Then I was so happy that I had new hair growing in. Well, now I have a topcoat and an undercoat!

My topcoat is dry, dull, brittle, faded, graying, and very thin. Super attractive! My new undercoat has grown in about four inches. It is very fine, soft, and CURLY! This new development has made it difficult to do anything with my hair. It is thicker on my head and much thinner hanging down. The new baby hairs are very unmanageable; most days they stick out all over my head doing their own thing.

Tonight, after speaking to the women's Bible study at our church, a young girl approached me and said, "Your hair looks really bad in front." Then she turned and walked away. My friend Samantha and I watched her leave, and then we both fell out laughing. It was a true statement. My hair has a life of its own right now. Her honesty made me smile. This crazy hair is proof of life to me!

Friday September 18, 2010

This afternoon we received a phone call from the oncologist's office with the report of my six-month PET scan - "All clear!" That's exactly what I was expecting, but it sure was nice to hear them say it. I am six months removed from chemotherapy, and there is no evidence of disease in my body. I can't even put my feelings into words at this point.

Recently I have been reading some of the old familiar stories in the Old Testament. I was studying the story of Noah the other day and read this verse: *"But God remembered Noah..."* Genesis 8:1 (NLT)

Isn't that beautiful? God remembered Noah. He remembered. And He remembers me too.

That simple verse should change how I think about situations in my life; it should change my actions and responses to life. God remembers me! How amazing is that? I'm pretty sure He was smiling, too, as the words "All clear" rang out over the phone. And God remembered Laura.

Tuesday September 21, 2010
Confirmation!

I had an appointment with my oncologist on Monday. After all this time, that still sounds weird. Who would ever think they would have an oncologist? I hadn't been to his office since June. It was so nice to see all the smiling faces and to receive hugs from everyone who works in his office. Mark asked me how I felt going in there, and I told him that I was just happy to be there as a "well" person and not as a "sick" person.

They weighed me, drew my blood, checked all my vital signs, and gave me a flu shot. The doctor did a thorough physical exam. And then he said to me, "Hit the road. I don't want to see you until December."

That is the third confirmation in a matter of days that I am healthy, I am healed. I feel such a profound joy, an indescribable lightness.

Later, when no one else was home, I went running, screaming, laughing, and dancing through the house! My God *is* an awesome God!

"I will thank you, Lord, among the people. I will sing your praises among the nations. For your unfailing love is higher than the heavens. Your faithfulness reaches to the clouds. Be exalted, O God, above the highest heavens. May your glory shine over all the earth." Psalm 108:3-5 (NLT)

Monday October 4, 2010
Sunrise

I have a t-shirt that says "Cancer Sucks" in big bold letters. Every time I wear it I get one of two responses from people who see it. They either look at me really weird, or they love the shirt and ask where I got it. I don't want to offend anyone, so I am careful where I wear the shirt. But the truth is cancer does suck. And now I am discovering that I need a new shirt, one that says "Cancer Recovery Sucks".

I felt really great right after I finished all of my treatment and surgery; so happy to be alive, so happy to be finished with treatment. Those feelings lasted for a while, and then slowly they settled into a darker place. The interesting thing is that the more I talk to other cancer survivors, I find that I am right on track with my thoughts and feelings. They've all been here too. They've all experienced the doubts and questions, the grief and confusion, the loneliness.

I read recently that about twenty-five percent of all cancer patients and survivors suffer from depression, and up to nineteen percent suffer from post-traumatic stress disorder. Those are big numbers. I'm pretty sure the same could be said of their family members too. I think it is important to be aware that depression often comes on the heels of a great victory.

Around 6:00 a.m. today I woke up to the sound of the smoke detector chirping, alerting me that the battery needed to be replaced. I was not too happy. I stumbled out of bed and went in search of a nine-volt battery in the dark. Of course, as is *always* the case, we didn't have any. Due to the way the system is designed, simply removing the battery will not stop the chirping. I sent Mark upstairs to sleep, but unfortunately by this time, the dog had decided that it was time for breakfast. Realizing that I was not going to get any more sleep, I got up and fed all the pets. I plopped down in the chair in the living room and stared out the window at the darkness. As I sat there, the sky began to get light and I watched a beautiful sunrise unfold. And God spoke to my heart, "I am still here with you. I will continue to walk with you. You are going to be OK."

It was such a powerful moment for me. Knowing that God woke me up, not the smoke detector! Knowing that He painted the sky specifically for me today to remind me of His presence and His faithfulness. Knowing that I am OK. My God is amazing; He is everything I need.

I am praying and trusting that the dark clouds of despair will give way to a clear and constant vision of God's presence, His faithfulness, and His goodness.

"The heavens proclaim the glory of God. The skies display his craftsmanship. Day after day they continue to speak; night after night they make him known. They speak without a sound or word; their voice is never heard. Yet their message has gone throughout the earth, and their words to all the world." Psalm 19:1-4 (NLT)

Wednesday October 6, 2010
Some Good News!

Every so often I spend time on the Internet reading about colorectal cancer. You would think I would be tired of the subject by now, but I find myself drawn to continue to learn as much as I can, hoping that somehow my knowledge will prevent recurrence! It's funny how the mind works.

Dr. Ralph Berberich said, in his book *Hit Below the Belt*, "Cancer is never really over unless you die, have an autopsy, and are shown to be cancer free, in which case it is of no interest to you. The passage of time simply reduces the chance of recurrence, but it never completely eliminates it."

I imagine that every cancer survivor, as some point, ponders the possibility of recurrence. How would that feel? What would I do? What would that mean? And then you shake those thoughts from your mind and try to go on living.

Studies of people with my initial diagnosis of stage three rectal cancer have shown that there is a fifty-eight percent survival rate at five years. Those odds don't really sound too positive. But just this week, on one of my regular Internet cancer searches, I came across some amazing news. New research published on August 25, 2010 in *The Lancet Oncology* journal has shown that patients with a diagnosis of stage three rectal cancer who were treated initially with radiation and oral chemotherapy; and whose cancer responded by dying off completely (which is my story) have an increased five-year survival rate from fifty-one percent to more than eighty-three percent. That's a jump of over thirty-two percentage points. That may sound like complete mumbo jumbo, but to me, it sounds like LIFE! That's crazy good news! In my opinion, it might as well be one hundred percent now. There is no chance this cancer is coming back!

As happy as this new report makes me feel, God reminds me that my life is not dependent on medical reports or even on five-year cancer survival rates. All along it has been dependent on Him - on *His* plans, on *His* timetable, on *His* grace. I've been free all along. Free to live.

Monday October 18, 2010
Go Gently

"Go gently through this day, keeping your eyes on me."
Sarah Young, *Jesus Calling*

I remember when our kids were little trying to teach them the meaning of the word gentle. Any time they were around babies or animals I would instruct them to be gentle or touch gently. The idea was to keep them, whether by enthusiasm or ignorance, from causing harm to others. I didn't want them to frighten young children by running over them, to harm babies by squashing them, or to overdo it when loving animals. It was something I found that had to be taught to excited, adventurous toddlers.

I remember once when David was two years old and Sarah was three months old, not knowing exactly how to play with his new baby sister, David decided to sit on her like a horse. I heard lots of squealing and laughter and I came around the corner to find him seated on Sarah's belly. Of course I panicked, screamed, and caused everyone else to start crying! David didn't realize the harm he could have caused his baby sister, Sarah was too small to defend herself as she struggled to breath, and I just exacerbated the situation by frightening everyone involved. This was the beginning of our life lessons in gentleness.

Today, I read the quote above in *Jesus Calling* by Sarah Young, and it just seemed to stick with me. How often do I go gently into my day? Have I *ever* gone gently into a new day? I guess in all those life lessons, I never applied the idea of gentleness to myself. So many times I go racing through the day. Sometimes I hurt other people because I forget to go gently. Sometimes I miss God completely because I forget to slow down and focus my eyes and thoughts on Him.

God reminded me today to go gently. Gentleness isn't just a lesson for toddlers. It's a better way to live.

"Take my yoke upon you. Let me teach you, because I am humble and gentle at heart, and you will find rest for your souls." Matthew 11:29 (NLT)

"But the wisdom from above is first of all pure. It is also peace loving, gentle at all times, and willing to yield to others. It is full of mercy and good deeds. It shows no favoritism and is always sincere." James 3:17 (NLT)

Saturday October 23, 2010
Conversations

Mark: "You better not die. If you die, I'll kill you!"
Me: "Oh, I'm not dying! I fought way too hard to live!"

Me: "I feel like I'm falling apart."
Mark: "Let's give it two years, two years to recover. And I'm just glad I have you for two years."

Me: "I feel really insecure. I feel weak. And it's so frustrating because I felt so strong before all of this.
Mark: "You are so incredibly strong, you just can't see it right now. When you come out the other side you are going to be amazed at what God has done!"

Me: "I feel like I've let you down. I feel like I'm a burden to you."
Mark: "You have never failed me. You are not a burden. You are the love of my life."

Mark: "I love your scars. They mean you're alive! You're with me. And I love your hair just like it is."

"Love never gives up, never loses faith, is always hopeful, and endures through every circumstance." 1 Corinthians 13:7 (NLT)

Monday November 1, 2010
Conversations Part 2

A man walks up, his face twisted with grief, and says, "My dad died of colon cancer." He hangs his head and walks out the door. (Spoken to me the day we announced my cancer to the church.)

"It wasn't the cancer that killed him, it was the chemotherapy." (Spoken to me the day before I started chemotherapy.)

"I've seen corpses that look better than you." (Seriously, someone said this out loud to a friend of mine who is fighting cancer!)

"You look tired." (Seems like an innocent statement. But please know that cancer patients are aware of how they look. They spend a lot of time trying not to look sick, but eventually, there is no hiding it. Please don't remind us. Unless you have a very close relationship with someone, don't make this statement.)

In the words of my mother (and probably yours too): "If you don't have anything nice to say, don't say anything at all." *"Words kill, words give life; they're either poison or fruit—you choose." Proverbs 18:21 (The Message)*

Friday November 5, 2010
Live Strong

I meet a lot of cancer survivors. They all seem to be doing well - big smiling faces, busy lives, no complaints. Every once in a while, one of them will quietly ask me, "How are you doing?" with concern in their eyes, as if they know there is more to this recovery process than anyone lets on. And I would have to agree.

Yes, I feel good. Yes, I am doing great. Yes, I am so thankful to be back to a normal life, whatever that means. But apparently when you are faced with the truth of your own mortality it has a deep impact on your psyche. At least it has on mine.

So God and I have been discussing these issues. Daily serious discussions like this:

Me: "What is wrong with me?"

Me: "Why can't I get over this?"

Me: "Why am I still thinking about this?"

Me: "Why do I feel this way?"

Me: "Why do I feel so insecure?"

Me: "I hate this."

God: (silence)

I persist, like He tells me to, in prayer. Asking for His wisdom. Waiting for His answers.

Slowly, I begin to move forward. I have (almost) whole days where I never even think about cancer, or at least not until the end of the day. And as the days pass, God begins to speak.

He reminds me that I am grieving, and grief is good. It is a healing process. It takes time. We all process grief differently, at different rates and in different ways. So I stop comparing myself to other cancer survivors. This is not, after all, a cancer survivor competition.

I realize that my insecurity is a grief reaction. I am afraid to go out and live my life strong because I am afraid that if I do, I might get slammed again, just like I did with the initial cancer diagnosis. It helps to see it for what it is. I am reminded of a book I read many years ago called *Feel The Fear And Do It Anyway*. So I decide to feel the fear and go ahead and live strong.

I am naturally a homebody. I love to travel, but when I am home I like to be at home. I don't have to go out and do things to be happy. I am happy at home. But over the last several weeks I have felt myself staying especially close to home. I have to force myself to get out every once in awhile just to go to the grocery store or run errands. Just this week I realized that this increasing need to hibernate is also a grief reaction. The world doesn't feel safe to me anymore. And so I hide away, trying to stay safe. It's strange how the mind works.

Today, I heard Nicole C. Mullen sing, and God's truth came flooding into my heart again:

"The very same God
That spins things in orbit
Runs to the weary, the worn and the weak
And the same gentle hands that hold me when I'm broken
They conquered death to bring me victory

Now I know, my Redeemer lives
I know my Redeemer lives
Let all creation testify
Let this life within me cry
I know My Redeemer lives"
("Redeemer," by Nicole C. Mullen)

And God speaks to me:
God: "I am still here with you."
God: "You are doing great!"
God: "Keep walking with Me. Live strong."
Me: "Thank You. I will."

"If you try to hang on to your life, you will lose it. But if you give up your life for my sake, you will save it." Matthew 16:25 (NLT)

Wednesday November 10, 2010
See You in Three Months

I have a new book: *Finding Your Way Through Cancer*, by Andrew Kneier. It was just recently published and recommended to me by a very sweet friend. The author is a psychologist who has worked with cancer patients and survivors for seventeen years. The book was written out of his experience with families affected by cancer.

I have just barely started reading the book, but one of the statements I read today hit home. It was from the journal of one of Dr. Kneier's patients who was fighting stage three colon cancer. She said this: "I get to live three months at a time."

That's what I'm doing. I'm living three months at a time. Three months between doctor visits where I wait for someone to tell me that I'm still healthy. So far, so good. No sign of the dreaded disease. Then they set another appointment for me and send me on my way. "See you in three months," they say.

Initially, I feel relief, I feel joy, I feel like laughing. I race home, let my family know, and get busy with life. But over the weeks, in barely noticeable increments, the anxiety starts to return. And as the end of that three months gets closer, I find myself starting to wonder again, "what if..."

It sure will be nice when I can live six months at a time.

Wednesday November 17, 2010
Reflections

"For we are God's handiwork, created in Christ Jesus to do good works, which God prepared in advance for us to do." Ephesians 2:10 (NIV)
The word translated "handiwork" in Greek is "poeima." It's the word for *poem*. "We are his poem." I like that. Our son David is a published poet. I'm saying that here not just because I'm proud of him, but also because having a poet in the family has helped me to understand this verse a little more clearly.

I have watched how David writes. He has ideas and thoughts in his mind, and it is almost as if they are alive in him. He *has* to write them down. And then he agonizes over the poem, crafting it just the way he wants it to be. He works for a while and then comes back to it later to rewrite a certain phrase or to change a word. He spends unbelievable amounts of time creating the poem to be exactly as he envisioned, so that it will express what is in his heart and mind, until finally it is finished. Then the poem is sent to the publisher and put on display.

I think that is what Paul is telling us in Ephesians. We are God's masterpiece, His workmanship, His poem. He is working in our lives to craft us to be exactly as He envisioned so that we will express what is in His heart and mind. He wants to display us to the world – as beautifully perfected masterpieces – each of us a demonstration of His power, His love, His character, His peace, His life. We are His poem.

God is working a masterpiece I might not always understand, but I can rest in the fact that He knows, He has a plan, and He is creating exactly what He desires in my life so that I will be a reflection of Him.

God, please let me be an accurate reflection of You today!

Tuesday November 23, 2010
My Life

The past ten days I've been busy working, planning, studying, shopping, running from one event to another, hosting friends, eating, laughing, and hanging out with family. I am completely exhausted, and completely content.

I was driving home the other day, tired all over, looking forward to climbing into my bed and putting the pillow over my head. Then I realized that these have been the busiest ten days I've had in the past eighteen months.

Do you know what that means?

My life is back to normal! I am not sick. This was my prayer and dream for so many months and my faithful God has given me what I dreamed. I have so much to be thankful for, it overwhelms me just to think about it all!

Sunday December 12, 2010
Solitary Road

There are days when I find myself still struggling. And then I find myself angry that I am still struggling. It seems like I should be able to pick up where I left off and go on with my life. But somehow things are different now. The path is unfamiliar and my steps are tentative.

I read the following quote from Elizabeth Edwards this week: "The act of looking forward after a setback is a solitary act…It is a gift, but also a learned skill…"

It describes perfectly how I feel - on a solitary road, learning a new skill, trying to recognize this as a gift from a God who knows perfectly what I need.

Tuesday December 28, 2010
Twisted Thoughts

Overcoming a life-threatening illness that has the potential to return kind of twists your thinking, at least it has mine. For example: "This cancer has the potential to return. If it returns it will be in my liver or my lungs. If it returns it will be worse. I will be even sicker. I will lose more weight. So I better hang onto the weight I have. Maybe I should gain a little extra. Just in case!"

Then one day I wake up and none of my clothes fit. They are too tight. I have gained back all the weight I lost during treatment, plus some. I share this with Mark, who says to me, "It might be time to quit the 'support package.'"

I laugh so hard at his comment, and I laugh at myself, at my silly thoughts. I guess it *is* time to do away with the support package and get back on the treadmill.

Friday January 21, 2011
New Pastime

Cancer produces a lot of side effects, and cancer treatment produces even more. Most of the side effects are short term or limited by the duration of treatment. However, there are some that are long term and require adjustments to be made as you live with them.

One of the most frustrating long-term side effects for me has been the loss of short-term memory. I recently read the following on my oncologist's website:

"Research has demonstrated that chemotherapy can have a negative impact on cognitive functioning. Long-term (5-year) cancer survivors who had received chemotherapy scored significantly lower on neuropsychological tests, particularly in the area of verbal memory, compared with those treated with local therapy only (i.e. surgery). The patients who received chemotherapy also reported greater problems with working memory and were more likely to score among the lowest on the Neuropsychological Performance Index. Furthermore, some survivors may experience long-term cognitive deficits associated with systemic chemotherapy."

Not very encouraging. And on top of that, researchers are not really sure of the actual cause of the memory loss and therefore have no helpful ways to treat it.

I recently asked my oncologist if there was anything I could do to help with the memory loss. He looked at me with his familiar shy smile and said, "I usually hand my patients a pad and a pen; but you are young, you can most likely re-train your brain." (I feel hopeful!) He recommended a trip to Target to pick up my new favorite pastime.

Doctor's orders: Play the Memory Game twice a day. Every day. This will help re-train the neurons responsible for short-term memory. In the meantime, write everything down.

Things I have learned in dealing with memory loss:
  1. Yes, Mark already told me, I just didn't remember.
  2. Make a list of the Christmas gifts you receive because you won't remember what you received or who you received it from when you sit down to write thank you notes.
  3. No, you won't remember, even when you think, "I'll remember this". Write it down.
  4. When a "good idea" comes to you, write it down immediately. Good ideas are fleeting and they may not come back.
  5. When speaking, always have notes; you won't remember what you were planning to say.
  6. ... Oops ... sorry, I forgot number six.

Tuesday January 25, 2011
Overload

At my last appointment with the oncologist, he asked how I was feeling. I told him that physically, I feel great, but emotionally, I am struggling. He assured me that this is normal. He said that this is the time frame when many cancer survivors experience a lot of tears. He said that I am suffering from post-traumatic stress. No surprise there! He also told me that it's OK not to be OK right now. Somehow those words bring relief to me. I'm right where I am expected to be.

I have read that because we have better treatments for many cancers now, more patients go on to live many years post treatment. While this is good news, it has also led to an increase in the number of cancer survivors experiencing post-traumatic stress and anxiety disorders. It has been reported that up to thirty-two percent of people will develop post-traumatic stress as a result of cancer diagnosis and treatment.

For me, it has led to moments of high anxiety where my body is physically shaking, days when I am very easily overwhelmed by life, feelings of anger that appear out of nowhere, and a heaviness that weighs on my heart from time to time.

I read these words this week:

"But blessed are those who trust in the Lord and have made the Lord their hope and confidence. They are like trees planted along a riverbank, with roots that reach deep into the water. Such trees are not bothered by the heat or worried by long months of drought. Their leaves stay green, and they never stop producing fruit." Jeremiah 17:7-8 (NLT)

I am reminded to reach deep, to soak in the Lord, to let His living water refresh me. I can never be overwhelmed because God is with me. He can't be overwhelmed.

Once again, His peace fills my soul, and I keep moving forward.

Sunday February 20, 2011
Abundant Life

Have you ever been reading the Bible and come across a verse you've read a thousand times, but for some reason this time God showed you something you'd never seen before? I had that experience last week.

I was reading in the book of John, in a different translation than I normally use, and came across John 10:10. I'd read it a thousand times before: *"I came that they may have life, and have it abundantly."* John 10:10 (NASB)

In the past, every time I'd read that verse I got stuck on the second half where it talks about abundant life. I wanted to know what abundant life is, do I have it, how do I get it, Every lesson I'd ever heard or read on that verse discussed the same thing.

But last week I saw something new. I hope I am able to explain it the way that God showed it to me that day. This verse is telling me what abundant life is and it's this: "I came..." Jesus came.

The fact that Jesus is here – His presence in my life – *that's* abundant life! It's not something else that I need to acquire, or something else I need to find or earn, or somehow get hold of. It's the presence of Jesus in my life – automatically I have abundant life. It's Him!

All throughout Scripture God uses the expression "I Am" to describe Himself. It means something that is happening in this present moment. He says I am the bread of life, I am the light of the world, I am the resurrection and the life, I am the way, the truth, the life, I am love, I am peace, I am strength, I am hope, I am... He becomes whatever we need in this present moment. That's the nature of who God is.

Jesus uses this same phrase here – "I am come..."

I am here, so you already have abundant life. You have everything you need. Abundant life is the opposite of overwhelming life. God was telling me to open my eyes and see that I already have abundant life in the midst of everything I am going through. There is nothing more I could ever possibly need because everything is met in His presence.

I remember when I was a kid in school. The atmosphere in the classroom was a certain way when the teacher was in the room and a different way when the teacher was out of the room. The teacher's presence made a difference in the classroom. Even if he just stood in the back of the room, didn't say a word, his presence changed everything. There was a power to his presence. Everything quieted down, every chaotic word or action fell into line, peace and order settled over the room. The teacher, by the authority of his position, was in complete control of the classroom.

That's what this verse in John 10 is saying. I am come. My presence in your life brings infinite love, and infinite power, and infinite wisdom. It brings peace, it brings rest, it brings hope, it brings order.

Consciousness of God's presence *is* abundant life. I need to constantly be aware of His presence with me. God is in my life; and He doesn't get overwhelmed.

Monday April 4, 2011
I Remember

This time last year I was wondering if the fear ever went away. I wondered if every PET scan and every lab test and every doctor's appointment would continue to bring up feelings of uncertainty. I wondered if there would ever come a day when I didn't think about cancer.

Well, last week I had PET scan #4, lab work, and a visit with the oncologist. Much to my surprise, I was not worried about the PET scan at all. I was not nervous waiting for the results. I didn't rehearse in my mind what I would do if the lab tests came back abnormal. In fact, when I walked into the doctor's office my heart was full of peace and confidence. I was so thankful to feel strong and well, and to be coming to his office as a healthy person and not someone who was signing in for treatment.

The doctor immediately came into the exam room, handed me my PET scan results and said, "Normal!" I think he was as excited as Mark and I were! He did a complete physical exam and declared me good to go for three more months. We stopped by the chemo infusion room to say hello to all the nurses who had become like family to us. There were lots of hugs and smiles all around.

As I left the doctor's office, Chris Tomlin's song, "I Lift My Hands" began to play in my mind again. The song has been in my heart ever since we first sang it at Community of Faith. But this day, the words were especially real for me:

"I lift my hands to believe again
You are my refuge you are my strength
As I pour out my heart these things I remember
You are faithful, God, forever"

God has been so incredibly faithful to me all my life, but I have seen it so clearly since that day I first heard the words, "You have cancer." And this day, *I remember, You are faithful, God, forever!*

I still think about cancer every day, but I consider that a good thing. Cancer occupies much of my daily prayer time as I intercede for so many friends and loved ones who are fighting this disease. But I am so happy to report that the fear and uncertainty are no longer a regular part of my daily life. *I lift my hands to believe again.*

Monday May 23, 2011
Give Me Faith

When I was in high school we lived in Southern California. One of the tourist attractions of the area was Disneyland. I made several trips to the happiest place on earth over the course of those years, enjoying all the rides, shows, and shops. The ride I remember best was called Space Mountain. It was a brand new roller coaster and the line to ride was hours long. After you finally boarded the ride and strapped yourself in, the roller coaster took off and you were plunged into pitch-blackness. The whole ride took place in the dark. There were invisible twists, turns, and drops. The blackness was pierced by screams and laughter. And when you came to the end, most people jumped off and ran to get in line to ride again. I was one of those people who loved roller coasters.

I guess maybe in some way those experiences helped prepare me for the whole cancer experience. Even after finishing treatment and going on to live my life, it still feels like I am on a roller coaster.

The highs include my own consistent medical exams and scans and friends' being declared cancer free. But the lows are heartbreaking; the shock of a family member diagnosed with stage four breast cancer, the discouragement of a good friend who has to endure her third surgery due to side effects of radiation, and grief, again, as another friend continues to struggle in his fight against colon cancer.

And on and on it goes.

Anger rears its ugly head again. I hate cancer. I hate that my family and friends have to deal with the grief, fear, pain, and complications of this disease. But even as I struggle with these emotions, God meets me there. I am sitting in the worship service at our church and we begin to sing:

> "I need you to soften my heart
> To break me apart
> I need you to open my eyes
> To see that you're shaping my life
> All I am, I surrender
>
> Give me faith to trust what you say
> That you're good and your love is great
> I'm broken inside, I give you my life
>
> I need you to soften my heart
> To break me apart
> I need you pierce through the dark
> And cleanse every part of me
>
> I may be weak
> But your Spirit's strong in me
> My flesh may fail
> My God you never will"
> ("Give Me Faith," by Mack Brock)

Tears come. God whispers to my heart: "Why are you so angry? You trusted Me in your own battle with cancer. Can you not trust that I am working in the life of your friends the same way?"

Will I trust You still?

"*Give me faith to trust what you say, that you're good and your love is great.*"

Wednesday August 10, 2011
God's Love Call

Living in the wake of cancer, at times I find myself still struggling
with residual thoughts and feelings. Thankfully, at this point,
it is not constantly on my mind, but most days it still enters my
thinking at some point. Not long ago, I spent the whole weekend,
several days in fact, despairing if I would ever find "me" again,
if anything would ever be the same again. Every thought, every
conversation, every waking moment was consumed by these
ideas.

And all weekend long there was a bird in our yard yelling at
me. He would swoop across the backyard squawking. He even sat
on the patio chair looking in through the back window – literally
for hours, without provocation – hollering at me, scolding me,
warning me.

I was aggravated. What is he doing? He is dirtying the chair!
Disturbing my peace!

Hours pass. The bird is still there – angry, determined,
frustrated, squawking. This bird is crazy! Everything is fine, the
yard is safe. We even *like* birds, for goodness sake!

The next morning I wake up, remember to spend time with
God, pray, journal, ask His forgiveness for trying to make it on my
own (again!) the last few days. I open up *Jesus Calling* for that day
and here is what it said (I kid you not!):

"As you listen to birds calling to one another, hear also my
love call to you… You can find me not only in beauty and
birdcalls, but also in tragedy and faces filled with grief. I can
take the deepest sorrow and weave it into a pattern for good."

God, it was You all along! Trying to get my attention, to pull my
focus back to You, to get my eyes on Your truth. You also gently

tell me that I have been sounding a little like that squawking bird – fussing, complaining and whining instead of resting and trusting in Your goodness. You're pretty funny! You can use anything and everything. You make me smile again. Thank You, Lord, for my crazy bird. And for never ceasing to call me, for never ceasing to meet me, for never ceasing to pull me up. Your love is never-ending. Please help me to recognize Your presence today in whatever form it takes! I love You!

"But ask the animals, and they will teach you, or ask the birds of the air, and they will tell you." Job 12:7 (NIV)

Tuesday August 16, 2011
Sweeter Than Honey

I had an appointment with the surgeon last week. As I sat in the waiting room I started thinking of all the things that had happened in the three months since I'd seen him last. I traveled to Africa, Costa Rica, Colorado, and Galveston; I enjoyed time with all my kids; I visited with all my extended family; our daughter Sarah got engaged; we bought a wedding dress; we baptized ninety-five people at our church, and we buried two friends.

As these thoughts swirled around in my mind, the voices of an elderly couple in the room broke through my thinking. They were there to see the doctor. She was obviously sick. And they were discussing the fact that this was the final road. They weren't upset. They weren't sad. In fact, they were happy, reminiscing about all the good things they had experienced together in their life. It was such a beautiful, peaceful, intimate conversation, I almost felt guilty for overhearing them. Such love. Such bravery. Such beauty.

I wondered to myself, when my time finally comes, will I face it with such grace and faith?

Once again I heard the words "All Clear!" from the surgeon. He congratulated me on the two-year anniversary of my initial surgery. He reminded me that we are going to continue to be aggressive in monitoring for any recurrence. I thanked him for that.

I walked to the car, fighting back tears of joy and gratitude for more time to live. Honestly, I wanted to shout it to the whole world: "I DON'T HAVE CANCER ANYMORE!"

Instead, I hopped in the car, sent an "All Clear" text message to Mark, and hit I-10 for the drive home. I turned on the radio and the words of "Even Now" by Will Reagan of United Pursuit began to play. They perfectly expressed the fullness of my heart:

"Your love is sweeter than honey, your love is stronger than

death, Your love lifts me out of my burdens, and shows me

how to dance."

Tuesday August 23, 2011
Continually

1 Thessalonians 5:16-18 tells us: *"Rejoice always, pray continually, give thanks in all circumstances; for this is God's will for you in Christ Jesus."* (NIV)

According to these verses God wants me to pray continually. He wants me to be full of joy, to give thanks all the time. I've heard that verse all my life, and my first thought is always, I can't do that. I can't do anything continually. How can I pray non-stop? That's ridiculous. And I skip over the verse.

This time I decided to study it more closely. By definition, the word "continually" means "without end or stopping, steady, or habitual." It is the picture of something that recurs frequently. A light comes on! God isn't saying that I have to be laughing and praying and giving thanks every second of my life; but He is saying that I should be doing these things so often that it appears that I never stop. That it seems to be without interruption. Suddenly, what God is asking me to do becomes possible.

Have you ever sat down at a piano keyboard and started playing a single note? You play it over and over and over until the sound seems to blend together, the sound of one note continues in the air until the next note is played. A hum begins to hang in the air until it sounds like there is no space in between the notes you are playing. It seems to be without interruption.

That's the picture the Bible is painting in this verse. My life should be characterized by joy, by prayer, by gratitude. So much so that it appears I never stop. One prayer should still be hanging in the air when I voice the next one. The result of my gratitude should still be felt when next I give thanks. My joyful smile should still be felt by one person when I share it with someone else.

That's what God wants me to do. Live my life like that. It brings Him pleasure and it brings me pleasure too.

Saturday September 3, 2011
Feeling Life

Have you ever really *felt* alive? *Felt* the strength and power living inside your physical body? Most of the time I just live my life, so used to living in this earth suit that I am not aware of the life that is present inside it. I go through the routines of my day without giving a second thought to the fact that there is *life* inside of me. Then I got sick with cancer. Suddenly, the fact that I had life, and that that life was threatened, brought it all clearly into focus. Each new morning was a celebration, every meal kept down a victory. The ability to take a walk or open a jar produced a wellspring of gratitude. Quiet moments, whispered prayers, unspoken looks became treasured proofs of life to hang on to.

Fast-forward two years.

I grab a walking stick and step into the river. The water is high, the current is strong. If I'm not careful, if I misstep, I will be quickly carried, tumbling, downstream. I plant each foot deliberately. I feel the strength of my thighs as I stand strong against the rapids. My heart is beating. Adrenaline is firing into my system. My lungs are drawing in clean, crisp mountain air. I follow my guide and begin to climb up over the falls to get to the quiet pools above. The river fights against my path; I struggle on, up over the giant rocks. Finally reaching the other side, I step on the rocks of the bank. I feel so alive. I feel so strong. And I begin to cry. I am so grateful for this moment. I am thankful that my body is healthy. I am thankful that I have *life* living in me. I am overwhelmed with gratitude. And so begins a private worship service, just me and my God. Feeling Life. You have been good to me!

"You gave me life and showed me your unfailing love. My life was preserved by your care." Job 10:12 (NLT)

Monday September 19, 2011
May I Please Be Excused?

Sunday evening, standing beside the kitchen sink, I slowly pour the Miralax powder into the glass, add water, and begin stirring. This is day five of twice-a-day laxatives shots, leading up to the full colon prep on Monday afternoon. Tuesday I have the pleasure of my fourth colonoscopy.

Miralax is colorless, odorless, tasteless and grit-less, but still I gag as it goes down. It's a conditioned response I'm sure. I make two batches of Jell-O, put apple juice and Sprite in the refrigerator. I am ready for Monday's clear liquid diet. I walk by the HalfLytely container. I can't even look at it. I dread the Monday evening adventure it implies.

I climb in bed Sunday night, thinking to myself, "God, may I please be excused?"

I remember as a child, coming in from playing outside, rushing through dinner, and then asking my mother, "May I please be excused?" I was finished with dinner and so ready to get back outside to play some more.

And I find myself with the same feelings. God, may I please be excused? I have done *everything* - all the treatments, and appointments, and surgeries, and lab work, and tests, and scans, and exams - I am *so* done with this! I want to go on. May I be excused? Please?

I'm sure He smiles at me. "Take My hand, Laura, let Me walk with you."

Monday morning. I am starving. My stomach keeps telling me to go fix something to eat. My brain intervenes (thankfully) and reminds me that Jell-O is the only thing on the menu today. I decide to make this as pleasant as possible and serve my Jell-O on Spode Christmas Tree china.

At noon I swallow a small pink tablet – Bisacodyl – it's stated purpose by the U.S. Food and Drug Administration is to cause diarrhea. Let the run – I mean *fun* – begin!

Are You sure I can't be excused yet, God?

Reading materials and baby wipes in the bathroom, check! Path cleared to the nearest bathroom (because I *will* be running!), check!

This evening's drinking of HalfLytely still blocked from my mind.

Wednesday September 21, 2011
Scanxiety

Scanxiety is a documented phenomenon experienced by cancer patients and survivors. The Community Dictionary defines it as "the tension which builds particularly amongst those who have or have had cancer as they move towards their regular check-up scan, hyperscanxiety being the period as they await results!" Luckily, I don't suffer from this phenomenon.

Tuesday morning, we are driving to the surgery center for my colonoscopy and Mark casually asks me, "So, how are you feeling?" "I feel fine," I reply. "I don't feel nervous at all."

And then I realize that in fact I don't feel *anything* at all. My emotions are completely shut down. What I *do* feel is tension in my jaw and knots in the muscles of my shoulders. I haven't slept well for a week. And it occurs to me that perhaps I am experiencing scanxiety, it's just manifesting itself in a different way than it normally does.

I ask Mark, "And how are you feeling?"

His answer, "I don't feel anything either. I'm numb."

Scanxiety victim number two.

The staff at the surgery center is amazing. I don't even feel the IV as it is inserted into my rolling vein. I climb onto the table, they gently cover me with a warm blanket (that I know will be stripped from my body as soon as I am asleep), I watch as two medications are injected into my IV, and that's the last thing I remember. I wake up in the recovery room to the sound of a sweet nurse, telling me that my colon is normal, handing me pictures of my insides, and telling me that the doctor will come see me soon.

My colon is normal. Did she just say that? I drift back to sleep.

A little later Mark and I arrive home. He wraps me in a giant hug and we hold onto each other, so thankful for good news one more time!

I feel like I can live again. At least for the couple more months until my next PET scan.

Wednesday September 28, 2011
The Perfect Dress

A few weeks ago Sarah, Ashley, and I set out on a search for the perfect wedding dress. We visited several wedding boutiques where Sarah was treated like the princess she has always been (hence the name Sarah!). After a two-day search, Sarah found the perfect dress and placed her order.

We were all excited and started the drive home. It's hard to believe that I really bought a wedding dress for my sweet Sarah! Every girl dreams about her wedding day, and it is so exciting to see those dreams come true for her.

On the way home, Sarah said, "Mom, I'm so glad you got to do this with me!"

I replied, "Of course I went with you! I wouldn't want to be anywhere else!"

Sarah paused and explained, "When you were sick, I didn't know if you would be here to do this with me." Her eyes filled up with tears and they spilled onto her rosy cheeks.

I started to cry too, so sorry for the fear my girl had to face, and so eternally grateful that I am here to be a part of her wedding.

Thank You, God, once again, for the gift of *this* day with my girls!

Monday October 3, 2011
Imagination

A year and a half after chemotherapy, I think I am doing well. Physically I feel great. Emotionally I seem to have conquered cancer. Spiritually I have learned so much more about my God. But then, out of the blue, it starts again.

Week before last, for two days, I feel tired. My immediate thought is that the cancer has returned. Anxiety takes over. I feel sick. I talk myself down. "You didn't sleep well for two nights. That is why you feel tired. Relax."

Last week, my stomach hurt. My immediate thought is recurrence. Then I remind myself that I just recently had a colonoscopy; my colon is healthy. I relax.

Today, I wake up with a headache behind my eye. My immediate thought is that the cancer has metastasized to my brain. I laugh at myself! "Really? Colon cancer doesn't normally go to the brain. It's just a headache. Relax."

It's tiring having an imagination!

Wednesday October 12, 2011
Today I Want to Acknowledge

I've been reading through the book of Romans in the New Testament. Just the other day I opened my Bible and picked up where I had been reading and this is what it said:

"Since these people refused even to think about God, he let their useless minds rule over them. That's why they do all sorts of indecent things. They are evil, wicked, and greedy, as well as mean in every possible way. They want what others have, and they murder, argue, cheat, and are hard to get along with. They gossip, say cruel things about others, and hate God. They are

proud, conceited, and boastful, always thinking up new ways to do evil. These people don't respect their parents. They are stupid, unreliable, and don't have any love or pity for others." Romans 1:28-31 (CEV)

I finished reading those verses and I sat there, deeply convicted that this is the most common lie I believe. I think I don't need God. And I live my life based on that belief. I don't think it consciously, but I operate as if that were the case.

Another translation of this verse starts with the words, *"Since they didn't bother to acknowledge God" (The Message).*

How often have I failed to even acknowledge God? Just started the day out on my own, gone to school or work without thinking about God? Tried to resolve issues on the job or struggles in my relationships without even acknowledging Him? How many times have I parented my kids on my own, without turning to God first? When I do that, I am basing my life on the lie that I don't need God, and that's a scary place to live.

The Bible very clearly tells me what the result of that belief is – if I refuse to acknowledge God in my life, my life will be characterized by these things: evil, wickedness, greed, indecency, gossip, cruelty, and pride.

And it's not complicated. God isn't asking me for something difficult. He just says acknowledge Me, think about Me. How do I acknowledge someone's presence? It can be as simple as a nod of the head, or a look in the eyes, but it changes how I operate, doesn't it? "I see you, I know You are here, I am living and moving and working with the knowledge of Your presence."

That's what God is saying. Think about Me, acknowledge Me in your life on a daily, moment-by-moment basis and as you do, you will naturally begin to live your life based on God's ideals and principles.

When I don't acknowledge my need for God on a regular basis, and I don't slow down long enough just to connect with God, to spend time with Him, to read and meditate on the Scripture, I am saying that I don't need God. "I've got this, God. No worries. I'm strong enough and smart enough, I have enough experience and good will to handle it. You go ahead and take care of other things."

And don't you know God's heart just breaks! "Not again, Laura, I've told you what's going to happen – wickedness, arguing, cheating, gossip, pride, stupidity..."

I've spent time with people who talk a lot about church, religion, and Christianity. They talk a good game. But I've also spent time with people who actually live what they are talking about. There is a big difference between the two.

James 1:26 says, *"Anyone who sets himself up as "religious" by talking a good game is self-deceived" (The Message).*

Christianity is not a religious belief system. It is intended to be a supernatural, personal relationship with the dynamic living God of the universe. That's what the Bible is talking about here, not just a nice, respectful belief system to help give me a peaceful, happy life. God intends for my relationship with Him to be life-changing, to be transformational, and to produce authenticity in me.

God, today I choose to acknowledge You. Thank You that You never leave me on my own. Thank You that I don't have to handle things by myself. Thank You that You are patient with me, constantly teaching me and waiting for me to get it. I love You for that!

Saturday October 29, 2011
He Knows

"The Lord is like a father to his children, tender and compassionate to those who fear him. For he knows how weak we are, he remembers we are only dust." Psalm 103:13-14 (NLT)

I have a weakness for pottery. I love the different shapes, the designs, the textures, the curves. I am intrigued by the fact that someone's hands formed the items I treasure, their creativity on display for others to enjoy. The bright colors bring me pleasure.

Whenever we travel, I usually find some sort of pot or vase to bring home as a reminder of the culture and country we visited. Many in my collection have been gifts from friends around the world, making them even more special to me.

One of my most prized possessions is probably the least expensive piece of pottery I have. Its value comes from the fact that it was given to me by my sweet Batwa friends in Burundi, Africa. They spent a week mixing the mud themselves, forming the pot, smoothing it with their hands, delicately carving designs around the side, and lovingly setting it in the fire to dry. They diligently worked together with me in mind, making gifts for all the guests who were coming. On the day of our final visit to their village, they thanked us for our friendship; they danced with us, prayed for us, and presented each of us with the gift of their handiwork. I was humbled and honored by their generosity.

I knew this piece of pottery was extremely fragile, and I desperately wanted it to survive the journey to my home. I carefully wrapped the pot in my clothing, filling the inside and wrapping several t-shirts around to protect it. I put it in my carry-on bag, placing things around it to keep it from bouncing around during the trip. I cushioned it above and below. I carried it with me in the car to the airport. I kept it in my hands all through the airport. It never left my sight, except as it passed through the x-ray machine at the security checkpoint. Even then, I was watching my bag go through the machine and I grabbed it as soon as it passed through. I kept it with me as we waited to board the plane, and I gently set it under the seat in front of me on the airplane. I kept my eye on it during all three flights home, making sure it didn't get bumped or roll around.

I knew that this pot was delicate. I knew that even an unintentional blow could shatter what was so special to me. And because I knew that, I took extreme measures to take extra special care of the pot. Thankfully, the pot made it home and is now proudly on display!

As I was reading Psalm 103:13-14 the other day, God reminded me of the Batwa pot. It's the picture of what God is saying in this verse. He knows how weak I am. He remembers that I am only dust. Just as I took extreme care of the fragile Batwa pot, God is lovingly caring for me. He wraps me up in His love. He fills me, He protects me. He never lets me out of His hands, and He never takes His eyes off me. He knows me, and so He carries me. I am grateful for a God who so lovingly "remembers we are only dust."

Wednesday November 30, 2011
Think Again

The cancer journey has been one of the most difficult experiences of my life. In the middle of it all, I read this in *Jesus Calling* one day:

"This is a time of abundance in your life. Your cup runneth over with blessings... I want you to enjoy to the full this time of ease and refreshment. I delight in providing it for you."

I literally laughed out loud. This had been the hardest time ever.

My reality had been rocked to the core. My family was shaken. I thought to myself, "Well, these words are off the mark today." This is certainly not a time of abundance and blessing and ease and refreshment.

Then God opened my eyes and spoke to my heart: "Laura, you are looking at it wrong. Your focus is off. These words are true. They are always true of your life, not based on your circumstances, but on My character."

God is still God. He is still on His throne. He is continually pouring out His blessing and abundance on me. He continually offers refreshment to me if I will look to Him to find it. He will ease the way if I let Him carry the burden. He promises to be strong in my weakness. He delights in providing for me!

What a change of thinking! What a profound turnaround of everything. The circumstances don't matter – they don't change the fact that my life is overflowing with God's goodness and blessing always, no matter how it may seem or how it may feel or how difficult it may be.

2 Chronicles 20 tells the story of King Jehoshaphat, my favorite story in Scripture. God performed an amazing miracle and turned what the enemy intended to be the destruction of God's people into a "Valley of Blessing." That's what God does! I can't wait to see all that God is going to do as He turns my cancer journey into a "Valley of Blessing" for me.

"Give thanks to the Lord; his faithful love endures forever."
2 Chronicles 20:21 (NLT)

Monday March 12, 2012
Get Your Rear in Gear!

Last weekend my friend, Teri, and I traveled to Tulsa, Oklahoma to participate in the *Get Your Rear In Gear 5K* with my daughter

Sarah and some of her friends.

In their own words, *Get Your Rear In Gear* "are sisters, brothers, mothers, fathers and friends who have been affected by colon cancer and want to do *something*." Their mission is to "Empower local communities to promote prevention and early detection of colon cancer and to provide support to those affected."

Teri and I arrived in Tulsa and immediately went to Runners World to pick up our race packets. We felt like athletes as we browsed through the store's running gear. In the back of my mind I wondered what I had gotten myself into. Yes, I ran track in sixth grade, but that was a long time ago!

We enjoyed a high-carb dinner at Olive Garden under the guise that our training required such extravagance. Then we spent the evening making t-shirts for our team (by that I mean Sarah spent the evening making t-shirts for our team).

The day was predicted to be cold and wet, but Saturday morning arrived beautiful, cool, and clear. We put on our running gear, loaded up the car and headed down to Veterans Park.

Sporting my "survivor" t-shirt, I stepped up to one of the tables to fill out a form in honor and memory of several of my sweet friends. As I was doing so, the lady at the table said, "Laura Shook! Is that you? I've read your story! I'm so glad you are here." It was another special moment to remember all those who prayed for me and championed me in the battle. It was the perfect inspiration to start the run.

The race route was beautiful, taking us over and along the river, winding through a peaceful tree-lined neighborhood and then back to Veteran's Park. Over five hundred people participated in the event, from age seven to ninety-nine!

It was a surreal experience to be running in a 5K almost three years after staring death in the face and being told that I had a 50-50 chance of survival. I took such pleasure in the sun reflecting off the river, the daffodils pushing up through the dirt, and the wind on my face. My heart was bursting with gratitude for life, for my family, for my friends, for my doctors, and for my faithful God.

One of the things that touched me the most was all the people I saw who were running in memory of their mothers and fathers – a sweet tribute to their loved ones, and the sad reality of the ugliness of cancer.

As Teri and I rounded the bend heading into the finish line, our friends were there cheering. Sarah ran out and joined us to cross the finish line together. Her smiling face beside me was my reward!

I am happy to report that we finished the 5K and we didn't come in last! Although "bringing up the rear" would have been totally appropriate given the nature of the race.

Tuesday November 27, 2012
The Most Wonderful Words

Two and a half years, to the day, since my cancer diagnosis. I sit in Dr. Campos' office in a white paper gown, seated on the exam table. Mark sits in the chair, head back, eyes closed. Dr. Campos finally walks into the room with my six-inch-thick chart, trailed by some new medical student who quietly leans against the wall, listening, watching, and learning.

And then he speaks the most wonderful words ever.

"You are completely normal! Your PET scan was clear; all your blood work is normal."

The most amazing joy starts deep inside me, fills me and spills onto my face. For the first time I honestly feel that I've been healed, that this is over. I feel free. I feel alive. I have a future. Anything is possible! I feel like laughing and running and dancing!

Instead, I thank Dr. Campos. We all agree that it was God at work through him. His face breaks into a broad smile. He tells me to come see him in six months then heads to the next exam room.

Alone, Mark and I look at each other with wide eyes and crazy grins. We give each other double high fives across the room. We leave his office, still in wonder at the goodness of God toward us. What a lot we have to celebrate and be thankful for! I text the kids, my family, and friends along the way. Congratulatory text messages flood my phone as joy spreads.

Thank You, Jesus, for healing, for grace, for walking with me, for Your joy overflowing! Please let me live every moment to bring praise and honor to You. Please show me how.

Monday December 5, 2012
In Every Way

Recently Mark and I had dinner with some good friends. As we were sitting around talking after dinner, my friend asked, "Laura, would you say that cancer changed your life?" Mark and I both laughed out loud, looked at each other, and immediately answered, "Absolutely!" And then she asked, "In what way would you say your life has been changed?"

The thought of it left me almost speechless. The change has been all encompassing. The only words I could speak were, "In *every* way." And those words seem so inadequate to describe what has happened. *Everything* about me is different. I may look the same on the outside, it may seem that my life has returned to the way things were, but the truth is that everything has changed.

The way I think, the things I think, the way I feel, the dreams I have, my relationships with family and friends, my relationship with God. There is *nothing* that has not been profoundly affected in some way. I am a completely different person on the inside.

And I wouldn't change it for the world.

I am stronger than I have ever been. I am more confident than I have ever been. It has caused me to speak my mind even more than I used to. I'm not sure that everyone else thinks this is a good thing, but I am very happy to do so!

I am not afraid of anything. I have an unshakeable peace. I know without a doubt that my life and my future are held in the hand of God. There is nothing that can come against me that God and I together can't handle. I know that He will always stand on my behalf. There is tremendous peace in the knowing.

My priorities have become more focused. I don't waste time or energy on things that don't fit into those priorities. Family matters. My friends matter. God's Kingdom matters. And that's about it.

I am constantly aware that life is fragile and death is certain. That may sound morbid, but honestly, it makes each moment sweeter because I recognize the gift and value of each day I am given.

So, yes, cancer changed my life. Completely. Thankfully.

Tuesday May 27, 2014
Five Years

I wake up today to praise music playing in my head. It's May 27th, 2014. Five years from my cancer diagnosis. I immediately begin to pray, thanking God for these five years, thanking Him for all He's taught me, and thanking Him for allowing me to know Him.

Nothing can take my joy away today. I am alive and I am healthy!

Five years ago today I was lying on a stretcher, having a colonoscopy for what I thought was hemorrhoids. What a difference a day can make! I woke up from anesthesia to find myself on a new path. A journey that I thought would be frightening and horrible, a journey that I didn't choose and didn't want. But it has turned out to be one of the most amazing experiences of my life.

I have met the kindest, most compassionate people ever. I have seen the goodness of God's people around the world. I have seen actual miracles take place. I have developed deeper relationships with my family. I have found the peace of God's presence. I have learned that when I am weak, He is strong, every time. I have discovered the freedom of giving up control. I know the joy of trust. I have no doubts about God – who He is or His word. My fears have been replaced with knowledge that whatever comes my way will be OK. The intimacy I have with my Savior is something I would never trade, not even for good health, as awesome as that is!

Thank You, God, for five years. Thank You for where we've been and what You have been teaching me. Thank You for allowing me to know You like this, for knowing that I am safe in Your arms, that You are totally and completely trustworthy. Thank You for showing me how strong I am and that we can do anything together. Thank You for all the new friends I have made along the way. Thank You for time alone together on the couch to pray. Thank You for teaching me to control my thinking and the power of my thoughts. Thank You for never leaving me, for walking with me every step of the way, every run to the bathroom, every tear-filled night, every screaming meltdown, every doubt, every angry outburst, every ride on a stretcher, every retch of my stomach. Thank You for calming every fear, for holding me.

There aren't enough words, so I'll stop here. I love You so much. Help me always to remember. Help me be as faithful as You are. Thank You for this unexpected gift of Your unfailing love. Thank You for teaching me to forever hope.

"Though the mountains be shaken and the hills be removed, yet my unfailing love for you will not be shaken nor my covenant of peace be removed," says the Lord, who has compassion on you." Isaiah 54:10 (NIV)

ACKNOWLEDGEMENTS

I would like to thank:

My doctors, Dr. J.R. Cali, Dr. Luis T. Campos, Dr. Neil E. Sherman, and their teams, for their compassion, dedication, and life-giving words. You made this possible.

My family who have always believed in me, and daily challenge me to be more than I ever dreamed possible.

Teri Leatherman, Erica Stidham, Nancy Miller, and Judy Aishman, who taught me the true meaning of friendship as they carried me through the "valley of the shadow of death."

Our staff and friends at Community of Faith, who walked the last five years with us, and never faltered in their belief that God would heal me. Your love and prayers give me life.

Kristy Stark and Lainie Thomas who wholeheartedly ran out all the details in order to complete this project. It wouldn't have happened without you.

Kelley Nikondeha for gently nudging me to finish what I started, for offering her constructive criticism, and cheering me along the way.

Melissa Lasater for faithfully praying each Monday and for making me laugh every day. You are a gift.

Dr. Todd Swift and the team at Maida Vale Publishing – especially my tireless typesetter Edwin Smet – for encouraging me to share my story and providing the way to do so.

This book is written in memory of those who never celebrated five years. "*It's been an honor to fight beside so noble a warrior and a great friend.*" C.S. Lewis

I DEDICATE THIS BOOK TO MY CHILDREN

I don't know if I've ever told you how much your encouragement, love, and support meant to me all through my cancer treatment and recovery; so that is the purpose of this note.

I know it was probably difficult for you to be so far away and not have the opportunity to follow things on a daily basis. In fact one of the hardest things for me was knowing that in some weird way I had caused suffering and grief for my family.

As I faced decisions about my treatment and my future, your faces were front and center in my mind. My choice to go forward with IV chemotherapy was based on my desire to live longer with you, and to see more of what God is going to do in your lives.

I carried your pictures with me to every radiation and chemotherapy treatment, and to every hospital stay. You were my inspiration. On the most difficult days, in the times when I was scared, and in the moments when I wondered if I could follow through with my treatments, I would pull your picture out of my Bible and remember – I had a purpose and a reason for enduring. You all gave me hope. The promise of more days and years with you gave me the strength I needed to persevere.

Your cards, emails, letters, texts, flowers, gifts, photos, phone calls, and visits brightened every moment.

Thank you for listening. Thank you for laughing with me and for crying with me. Thank you for playing games with me. Thank you for always looking on the positive side of things. Thank you for all the things you did to help me. Thank you for understanding when my feelings and emotions were out of whack. And thank you from the bottom of my heart for encouraging and supporting your daddy through it all.

I am so proud to be your mother and to call you my children. Each of you is so incredibly amazing! I love how you pursue your dreams. I love how you strive to make a difference in the world, and how you allow God to use you to do so.

We've made it through the first five years. We don't know what the future holds, but I do know that God is good and His plans for us are good. I pray you will never doubt that.

I love each of you with all my heart. Thank you for walking with me on this journey.

YOUR HEALTH IS IN YOUR HANDS

The American Cancer Society reports that half of all men will develop some form of cancer in their lifetime and one third of all women. You can be diagnosed at any age. Cancer isn't just a disease of the elderly anymore. The incidence of many forms of cancer is increasing in young adults.

Only five percent of all cancers are hereditary, meaning that the rest can be prevented with lifestyle changes or early detection and treatment. Breast, Colon, Rectal, Oral, Skin, Cervical, Lung, Prostate, and Testicular cancer are all either preventable or very treatable when caught early. So, take charge; your health is in your hands!

Eat well. Be active. Don't smoke. Get screened.

If you are a woman:
- Do monthly self breast exams
- Get an annual physical and pap smear
- If you are over age 40 get a mammogram
- If you are over age 50 get a colonoscopy
- Use sunscreen daily

If you are a man:
- Do monthly testicular exams
- Get an annual physical
- Remember men get breast cancer too
- If you are over age 50 get a colonoscopy
- Use sunscreen daily

If you notice changes in your health, trust your instincts, see your doctor. Keep pursuing the issue until it is resolved. You know your body best.

Your health is in your hands.

Colorectal Cancer

Most cases of colorectal cancer are preventable and treatable. If caught early, colorectal cancer is curable. Unfortunately, most cases of colorectal cancer are not discovered early. Early stages do not usually present with symptoms, which is why screening for colorectal cancer is so important. A colonoscopy could save your life by removing polyps before they become cancerous.

The following are considered risk factors for colorectal cancer:
> Over the age of fifty
> Use of tobacco
> Obesity
> Sedentary lifestyle
> Personal or family history of colorectal cancer
> Personal or family history of benign colorectal polyps
> Personal or family history of inflammatory bowel disease
> Family history of inherited colorectal cancer

To reduce your risk of colorectal cancer, exercise regularly, maintain a healthy weight, eat a high-fiber diet, don't use tobacco, and drink alcohol in moderation.

If you experience any of the following symptoms, no matter your age, see your doctor and get screened for colorectal cancer:
> A change in your normal bowel habits
> Excessive gas
> Constipation
> Diarrhea
> Alternating constipation and diarrhea
> Feeling that the bowel does not empty
> Bright red or dark red blood in the stool

Stools that are thinner than normal
Ongoing stomach discomfort
Excessive bloating, fullness or cramps
Unintentional weight loss
Loss of appetite
Vomiting
Constant fatigue
Anemia
Jaundice

For more information
American Cancer Society, www.cancer.org

American College of Gastroenterology, www.acg.gi.org

Centers for Disease Control and Prevention, www.cdc.gov

C3: Colorectal Cancer Coalition, (877) 427-2111,
www.fightcolorectalcancer.org

Colon Cancer Alliance, (877) 422-2030, www.ccalliance.org

National Cancer Institute, (800) 422-6237, www.cancer.gov

Prevent Cancer Foundation, www.preventcancer.org

Laura Shook has a heart that bridges oceans and cultures. After serving nearly a decade as a missionary in Mexico, she returned to Houston, Texas, where she founded Community of Faith with her husband Mark and three children. In ten years the church has grown to over 8,000 people in worship and has been listed among the top 100 churches in the country. Laura encourages people in Houston and around the world, and sets the tone for the international ministries of the church, as a tireless advocate for the broken and forgotten. Laura is a gifted speaker and teacher. She is a graduate of Baylor University and is a Registered Nurse. A cancer survivor, Laura lives each day committed to loving people and living full-out for Christ.

Forever Hope, an adaptation of her popular online diary, recounts the story of her journey from diagnosis to recovery in words full of wit, song, praise and everyday humanity. Beyond being a book simply for those who may be in treatment or recovery from cancer, this is a timeless memoir of how one should live daily with hope, love, good humor, and faith in a compassionate God, and is destined to be an inspirational touchstone for years to come.